The Complete Low Cholesterol Cookbook for Beginners

1500 Days of Nutrient-Packed and Heartwarming Recipes with a 28-Day Meal Plan to Promote a Balanced Lifestyle| Full Color Edition

Robin K. Solis

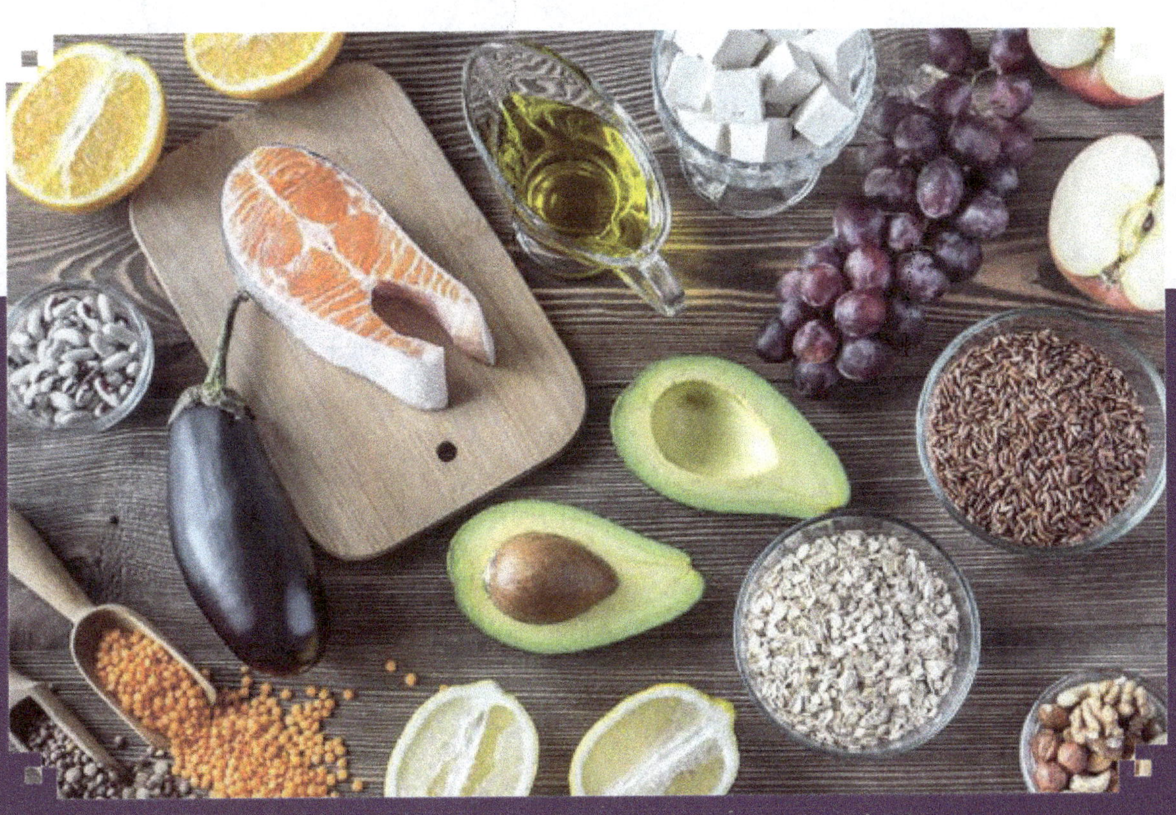

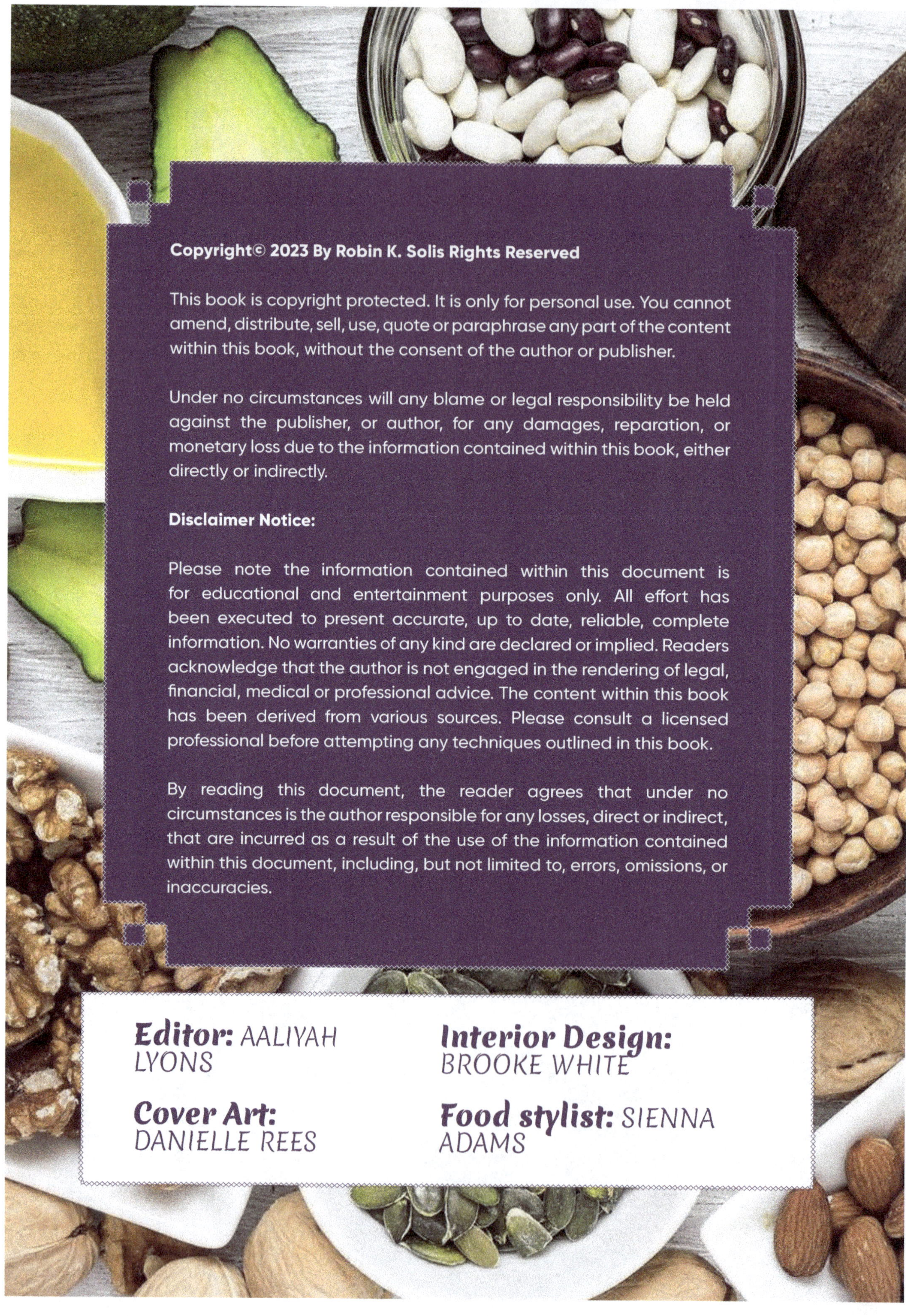

Editor: AALIYAH LYONS

Interior Design: BROOKE WHITE

Cover Art: DANIELLE REES

Food stylist: SIENNA ADAMS

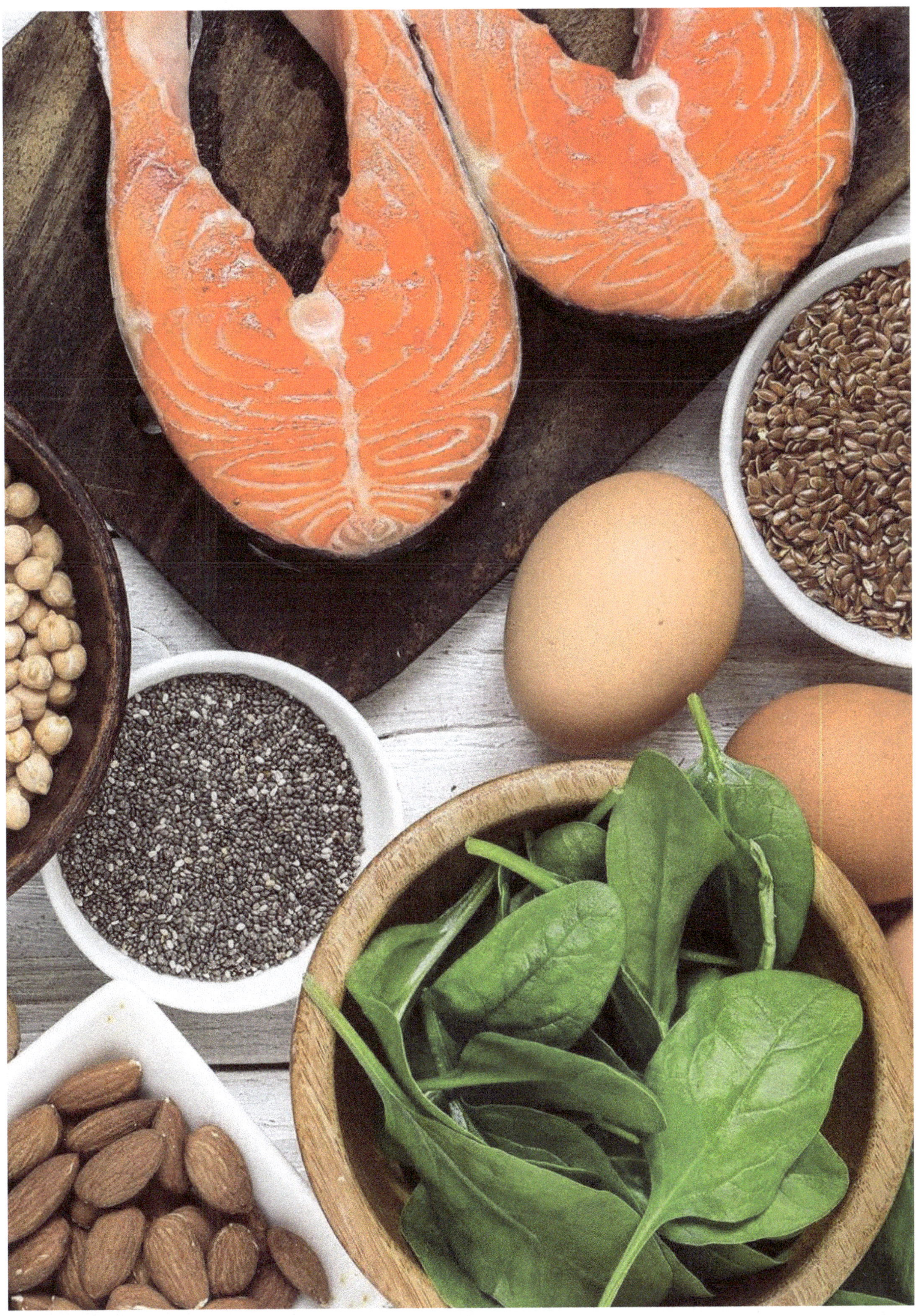

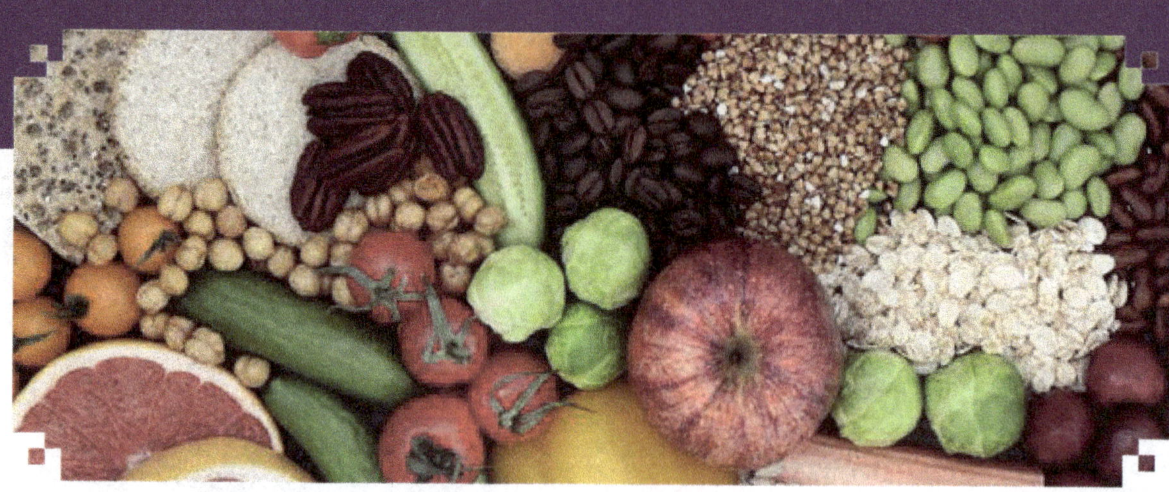

Table Of Contents

Introduction

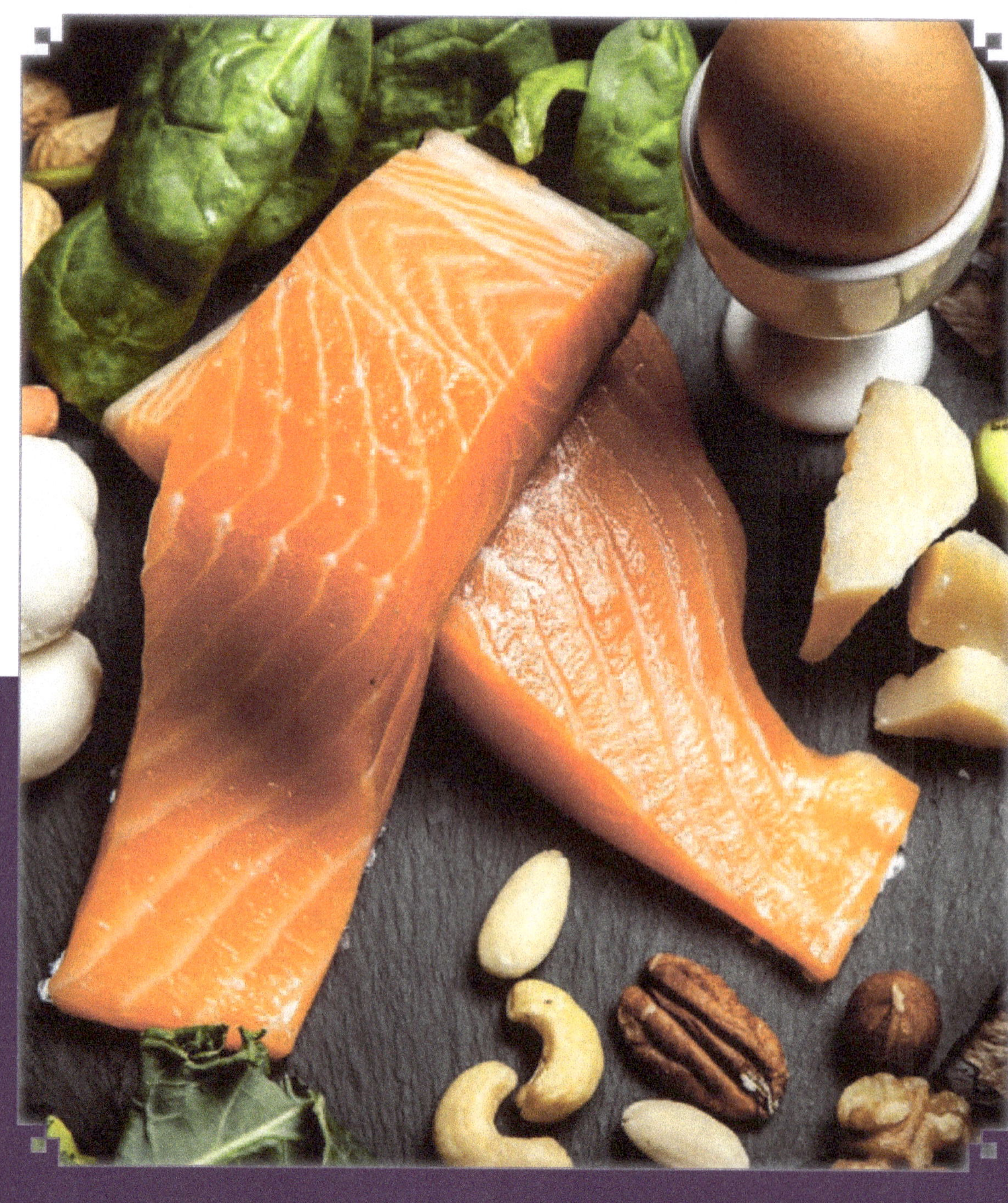

In the bustling landscape of modern life, where convenience often reigns supreme, our dietary choices play a pivotal role in shaping our well-being. With the increasing prevalence of lifestyle-related diseases, adopting a heart-healthy approach to cooking and eating has become more important than ever.

This cookbook is a labor of love, carefully crafted to empower you with delicious and nutritious recipes that not only tantalize your taste buds but also prioritize your cardiovascular health. In a world where fast food and processed ingredients often dominate our plates, this collection of culinary creations aims to show that eating for heart health doesn't mean sacrificing flavor or enjoyment.

In the following pages, you will embark on a culinary journey that fuses together the art of cooking with the science of nutrition. We've curated a diverse selection of dishes, from breakfast to dinner and everything in between, all designed to keep your cholesterol levels in check while delivering the satisfaction that comes with a well-prepared meal. Our team of expert chefs, nutritionists, and healthcare professionals have collaborated to ensure that each recipe not only adheres to the principles of heart-healthy eating but also delights your senses.

The importance of maintaining healthy cholesterol levels cannot be overstated. High cholesterol levels can lead to the buildup of plaque in your arteries, increasing the risk of heart disease and other cardiovascular complications. By embracing the principles outlined in this cookbook, you're taking a proactive step toward safeguarding your heart and overall well-being. But this isn't just about avoiding certain foods; it's about embracing a positive and delicious approach to nourishing your body.

While the recipes in this book focus on low cholesterol ingredients and preparation methods, they also celebrate the joy of cooking and sharing meals with loved ones. Food has the remarkable ability to bring people together, and we hope that these recipes not only become a staple in your kitchen but also inspire you to gather and create meaningful memories with those around you.

As you embark on this culinary adventure, take a moment to appreciate the ingredients that nature provides. Explore the vibrant colors, rich textures, and diverse flavors that contribute to the world of heart-healthy cuisine. From the fresh produce that graces your salads to the hearty grains that form the foundation of your entrées, every ingredient plays a role in promoting your well-being.

Remember that every small step counts. Whether you're a seasoned chef or a novice in the kitchen, the recipes in this cookbook are designed to be approachable and adaptable to your lifestyle. Feel free to experiment, modify, and make these dishes your own. Cooking is an art that allows for creative expression, and we encourage you to embrace the process with an open heart and a curious palate.

May these recipes not only nourish your body but also inspire you to cultivate a deeper connection with the food you eat and the impact it has on your health. Here's to a vibrant, flavorful, and heart-healthy life!

Chapter 1

Cholesterol and Your Health

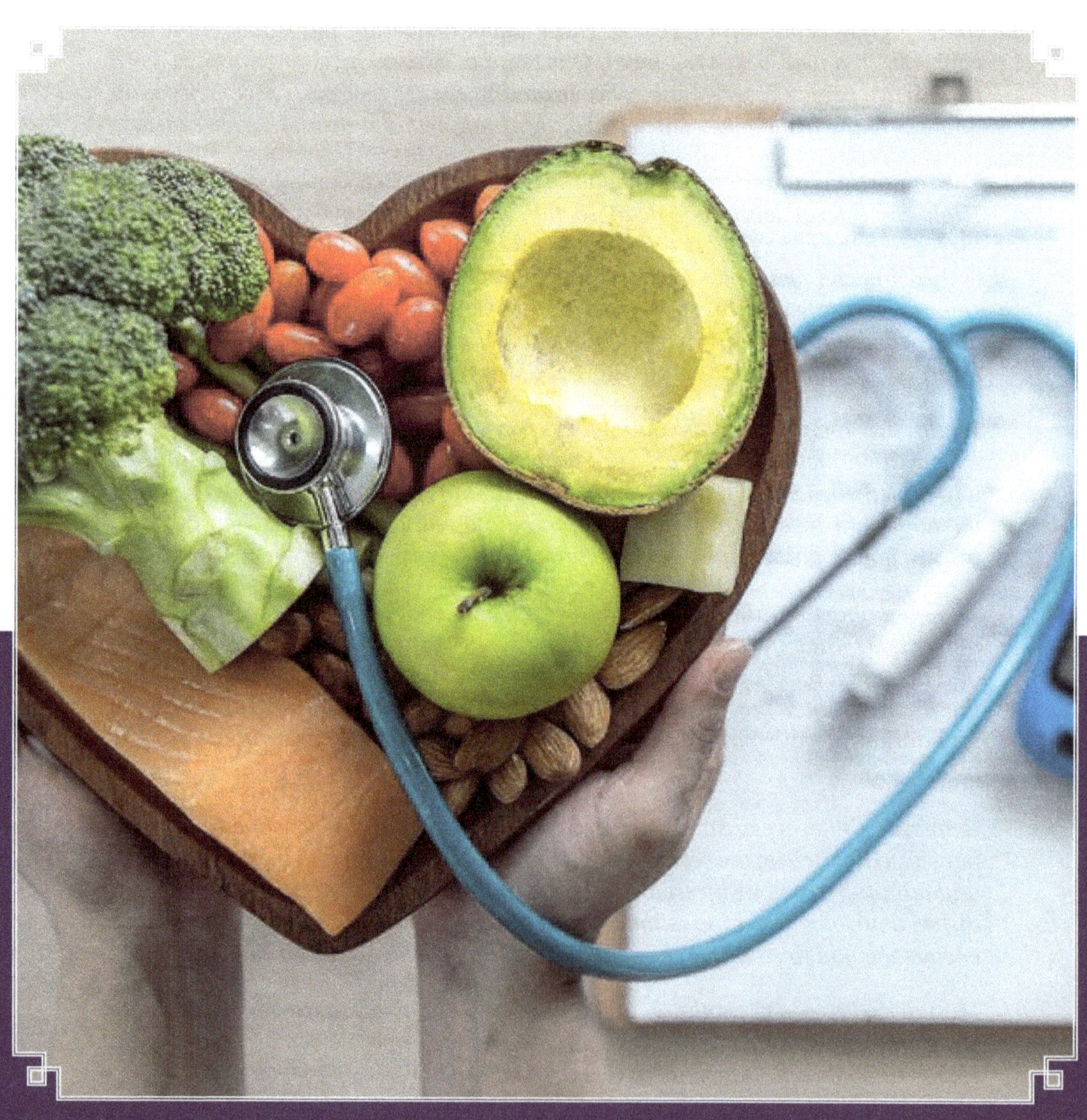

Know Your Cholesterol

In the realm of cardiovascular well-being, understanding cholesterol is akin to wielding a compass on a journey of optimal health. Cholesterol, often mentioned in hushed tones as a harbinger of heart ailments, is in fact an essential lipid molecule vital for various bodily functions. Grasping the nuances of cholesterol, differentiating between its types, and recognizing its implications is an empowering step toward taking charge of your heart health.

Cholesterol is a waxy, fat-like substance that is found in every cell of your body. It's not inherently villainous; rather, it serves as a structural component of cell membranes and acts as a precursor to hormones, vitamin D, and bile acids that aid digestion. However, the balance can tip when cholesterol levels soar beyond what the body requires. This excess cholesterol can accumulate within arteries, leading to the formation of plaques that narrow and harden the arterial walls, a condition known as atherosclerosis.

When discussing cholesterol, the focus often zeroes in on two distinct types: low-density lipoprotein (LDL) cholesterol and high-density lipoprotein (HDL) cholesterol. LDL cholesterol, often referred to as "bad" cholesterol, is responsible for ferrying cholesterol from the liver to cells, where it can accumulate if not properly managed. High levels of LDL cholesterol are linked to the development of atherosclerosis and an increased risk of heart disease. On the other hand, HDL cholesterol, often hailed as "good" cholesterol, scavenges excess cholesterol from cells and returns it to the liver for elimination. Higher levels of HDL cholesterol are associated with a reduced risk of heart disease.

Knowing your cholesterol levels is pivotal. Regular cholesterol checks, often done through blood tests, provide a snapshot of your LDL and HDL cholesterol levels, allowing you to monitor your heart health status. Ideally, your LDL cholesterol should be kept at lower levels, while higher levels of HDL cholesterol are desirable. Various factors influence your cholesterol levels, including genetics, diet, physical activity, and overall lifestyle.

In the grand tapestry of heart health, education and awareness are your allies. Armed with the knowledge of cholesterol and its nuances, you can make informed decisions about your dietary choices and lifestyle habits. A balanced diet rich in fiber, healthy fats, and whole grains can help manage cholesterol levels. Engaging in regular physical activity and avoiding smoking are also instrumental in maintaining optimal cholesterol balance.

Remember, the story of cholesterol is not one of absolute condemnation but of equilibrium. Understanding the roles of LDL and HDL cholesterol and their delicate balance provides you with a script to rewrite your heart's narrative. By knowing your cholesterol levels, making conscious dietary choices, and embracing a heart-healthy lifestyle, you're taking a significant stride toward nurturing your cardiovascular well-being. It's a journey marked by empowerment, one where knowledge becomes a guiding light on the path to a healthier heart and a fuller life.

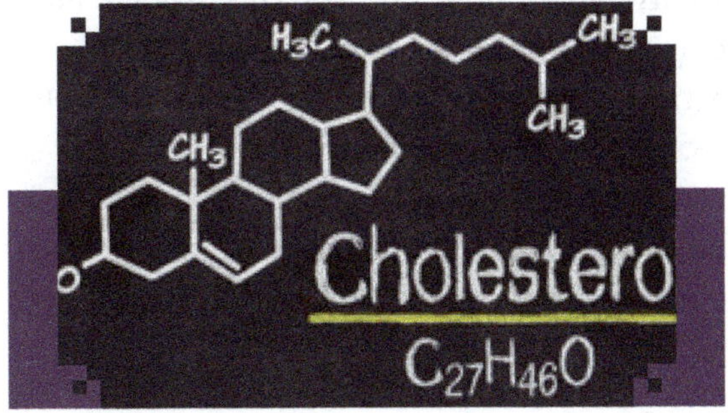

Types of Cholesterol

In the intricate landscape of cardiovascular health, cholesterol takes center stage as both a vital molecule and a potential health risk. Cholesterol, a type of lipid or fat, is indispensable for various physiological functions, but it also becomes a concern when its levels exceed the body's needs. To navigate this multifaceted subject, it's essential to comprehend the two primary types of cholesterol: Low-Density Lipoprotein (LDL) cholesterol and High-Density Lipoprotein (HDL) cholesterol.

LOW-DENSITY LIPOPROTEIN (LDL) CHOLESTEROL: THE CULPRIT BEHIND ATHEROSCLEROSIS

Often referred to as the "bad" cholesterol, LDL cholesterol plays a significant role in the formation of atherosclerosis—a condition characterized by the buildup of fatty deposits in the arteries. LDL cholesterol particles transport cholesterol from the liver to cells throughout the body, providing necessary lipids for cell membranes and various physiological processes. However, when LDL cholesterol levels surge beyond the body's requirements, problems arise.
LDL cholesterol particles can become oxidized, a process that renders them more reactive and capable of triggering inflammation within the arterial walls. In response to this inflammation, the body's immune system mounts a defense, sending white blood cells to the site. These cells engulf the oxidized LDL particles and form fatty plaques along the arterial walls, leading to the narrowing and hardening of the arteries. This process restricts blood flow, potentially leading to serious cardiovascular complications such as heart attacks and strokes.

HIGH-DENSITY LIPOPROTEIN (HDL) CHOLESTEROL: THE GUARDIAN OF CARDIOVASCULAR HEALTH

HDL cholesterol, often referred to as the "good" cholesterol, operates in stark contrast to its LDL counterpart. HDL cholesterol particles serve as the body's cleanup crew, removing excess cholesterol from cells and arterial walls, and transporting it back to the liver for elimination from the body. This scavenging action prevents the accumulation of cholesterol within the arteries and contributes to the maintenance of healthy blood vessel function.Beyond its cholesterol transport role, HDL cholesterol exerts other protective effects. It possesses anti-inflammatory and antioxidant properties, further guarding against the development of atherosclerosis. A high level of HDL cholesterol is associated with a lower risk of heart disease, making it a valuable component of cardiovascular health.

THE BALANCING ACT: LDL TO HDL RATIO AND TOTAL CHOLESTEROL LEVELS

While understanding LDL and HDL cholesterol individually is crucial, assessing their interplay provides a more comprehensive view of cardiovascular health. The ratio of LDL cholesterol to HDL cholesterol is an important marker that can offer insights into your risk of heart disease. A higher ratio suggests an increased risk, while a lower ratio indicates a healthier cardiovascular profile. Total cholesterol levels, which include both LDL and HDL cholesterol, are another key aspect to consider. Aiming for an optimal total cholesterol level is recommended to maintain heart health. However, this number alone may not provide a complete picture, as the balance between LDL and HDL cholesterol is equally important.

FACTORS INFLUENCING CHOLESTEROL LEVELS

A myriad of factors influences your cholesterol levels, some of which are within your control, while others are determined by genetics and underlying health conditions. Diet plays a pivotal role: consuming saturated and trans fats can elevate LDL cholesterol levels, while consuming unsaturated fats, fiber-rich foods, and plant-based sources of protein can positively impact both LDL and HDL cholesterol.Physical activity also plays a crucial role in managing cholesterol levels. Regular exercise can boost HDL cholesterol while promoting overall cardiovascular fitness. Weight management, smoking cessation, and limiting alcohol intake are additional lifestyle factors that can contribute to a healthier cholesterol profile.

Normal Cholesterol Levels

Cholesterol, often labeled as both a friend and foe to cardiovascular health, demands careful consideration and management. Recognizing what constitutes normal cholesterol levels is a fundamental step toward protecting your heart and preventing potential health complications. Let's delve into the intricacies of these cholesterol benchmarks and their significance in maintaining optimal well-being.

CHOLESTEROL LEVEL COMPONENTS

When discussing cholesterol levels, it's essential to focus on three primary components:

- Total Cholesterol: This encompasses the sum of various cholesterol types present in your bloodstream, including both Low-Density Lipoprotein (LDL) cholesterol and High-Density Lipoprotein (HDL) cholesterol. Monitoring your total cholesterol provides an overview of your cholesterol profile.

- LDL Cholesterol: Often referred to as "bad" cholesterol, LDL cholesterol is associated with an increased risk of atherosclerosis and heart disease. Elevated levels of LDL cholesterol can lead to the accumulation of plaque within arterial walls, potentially hindering blood flow and increasing the likelihood of cardiovascular events.

- HDL Cholesterol: Dubbed the "good" cholesterol, HDL cholesterol plays a protective role by removing excess cholesterol from arterial walls and transporting it to the liver for disposal. Higher levels of HDL cholesterol are associated with a reduced risk of heart disease.

NORMAL CHOLESTEROL LEVELS: GUIDELINES AND INTERPRETATION

The guidelines for what constitutes normal cholesterol levels have evolved over the years due to advancing research and understanding of cardiovascular health. As of my last knowledge update in September 2021, the following guidelines are generally considered:

- Total Cholesterol: A total cholesterol level below 200 milligrams per deciliter (mg/dL) is typically considered desirable. However, this number is best interpreted in conjunction with other factors, such as your LDL and HDL cholesterol levels.

- LDL Cholesterol: Optimal LDL cholesterol levels are generally less than 100 mg/dL. However, the interpretation can vary based on individual risk factors. For those at higher risk of heart disease, the recommended LDL cholesterol level may be even lower.

- HDL Cholesterol: HDL cholesterol levels greater than 60 mg/dL are often associated with a reduced risk of heart disease. A level below 40 mg/dL for men and below 50 mg/dL for women is considered low and may increase cardiovascular risk.

It's important to note that these values are guidelines and not absolute thresholds. Your healthcare provider will consider your overall health, medical history, and other risk factors when interpreting your cholesterol levels. Additionally, while cholesterol levels provide valuable insights, they are just one piece of the puzzle. Other factors, such as blood pressure, family history, and lifestyle habits, also contribute to your overall cardiovascular risk.

PERSONALIZED APPROACH TO HEART HEALTH

Cholesterol management is not a one-size-fits-all endeavor. A personalized approach, taking into account your individual health profile, is essential. If your cholesterol levels are not within the desired range, your healthcare provider may recommend lifestyle modifications, dietary changes, increased physical activity, and, in some cases, medication to help bring your levels into a healthier range.

Regular monitoring and open communication with your healthcare provider are crucial. Cholesterol levels can fluctuate, and adjustments may be needed to maintain optimal heart health. Remember that achieving and maintaining normal cholesterol levels is a journey that requires commitment and consistency, but the rewards are immeasurable—a healthier heart and a greater chance of enjoying a vibrant and active life.

Risk Factors of High Cholesterol

High cholesterol, often referred to as a silent menace, poses a significant risk to cardiovascular health. While cholesterol is essential for bodily functions, elevated levels of certain types can lead to atherosclerosis and heart disease. Understanding the risk factors associated with high cholesterol is a pivotal step in proactively protecting your heart and overall well-being.

GENETICS: THE INHERITED INFLUENCE

Genetics plays a notable role in your cholesterol levels. A family history of high cholesterol can significantly increase your risk. If close relatives, such as parents or siblings, have been diagnosed with high cholesterol or have experienced cardiovascular events, you may be genetically predisposed to elevated cholesterol levels. Genetic factors can influence how your body produces, processes, and clears cholesterol, making vigilance all the more crucial.

DIETARY HABITS: YOU ARE WHAT YOU CONSUME

The foods you choose to consume have a direct impact on your cholesterol levels. Diets rich in saturated and trans fats, commonly found in fried foods, processed snacks, and fatty meats, can elevate LDL cholesterol—the "bad" cholesterol—levels. Additionally, excessive intake of dietary cholesterol, often found in animal products like eggs and dairy, can contribute to elevated cholesterol levels in some individuals.

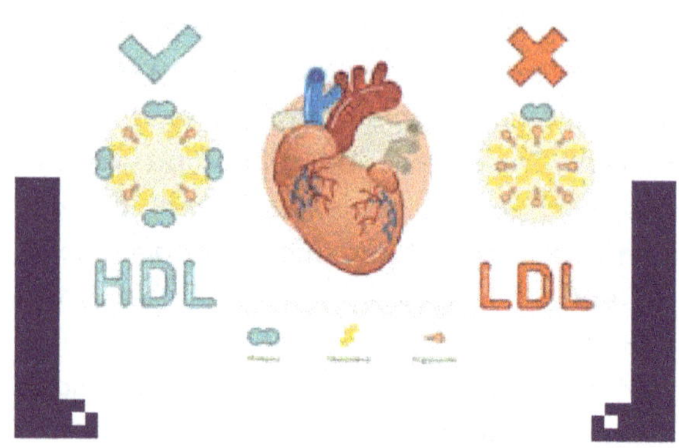

On the flip side, a diet high in fiber, whole grains, fruits, vegetables, and healthy fats—such as those found in nuts, seeds, and fatty fish—can promote healthier cholesterol levels. Fiber helps lower LDL cholesterol by binding to it and aiding its removal from the body. Dietary choices wield substantial power in influencing your cholesterol profile.

PHYSICAL INACTIVITY: THE SEDENTARY SEDUCTION

Lack of regular physical activity is a risk factor for high cholesterol and cardiovascular disease. Engaging in regular exercise helps raise levels of HDL cholesterol—the "good" cholesterol—which aids in removing excess cholesterol from arterial walls. Physical activity also contributes to weight management, and maintaining a healthy weight can positively impact cholesterol levels.

WEIGHT MANAGEMENT: THE BALANCING ACT

Excess body weight, particularly abdominal obesity, is linked to higher levels of LDL cholesterol and lower levels of HDL cholesterol. Obesity can also contribute to inflammation, which plays a role in the development of atherosclerosis. Losing weight through a combination of a balanced diet and regular exercise can help improve your cholesterol profile and overall cardiovascular health.

SMOKING: INHALING RISK

Smoking damages blood vessels and accelerates atherosclerosis. It lowers levels of HDL cholesterol while promoting oxidative stress, inflammation, and the formation of blood clots. All of these factors significantly increase the risk of heart disease. Quitting smoking is a crucial step toward improving your cardiovascular health and reducing your risk of high cholesterol-related complications.

AGE AND GENDER: INEVITABILITIES AND DISPARITIES

As you age, your risk of high cholesterol increases. This is partly due to changes in hormone levels and metabolism. Men generally have higher cholesterol levels than premenopausal women. However, after menopause, women's cholesterol levels tend to rise and often equal or surpass those of men. Age and gender are non-modifiable risk factors, but their awareness can encourage proactive health management.

DIABETES: THE INTRICATE CONNECTION

Diabetes and high cholesterol are interconnected health concerns. People with diabetes often have elevated triglyceride levels and lower levels of HDL cholesterol. Additionally, diabetes can damage blood vessels, making them more susceptible to cholesterol buildup. Managing blood sugar levels through medication, diet, and lifestyle changes is essential for maintaining heart health in individuals with diabetes.

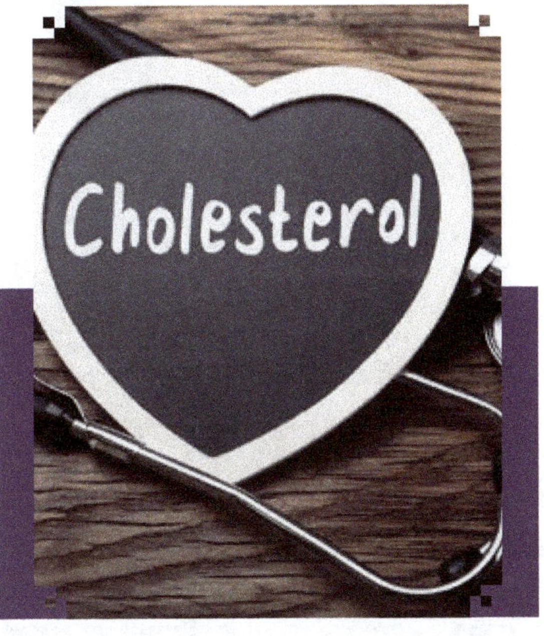

Chapter 2

Cooking in Your Low-Cholesterol Kitchen

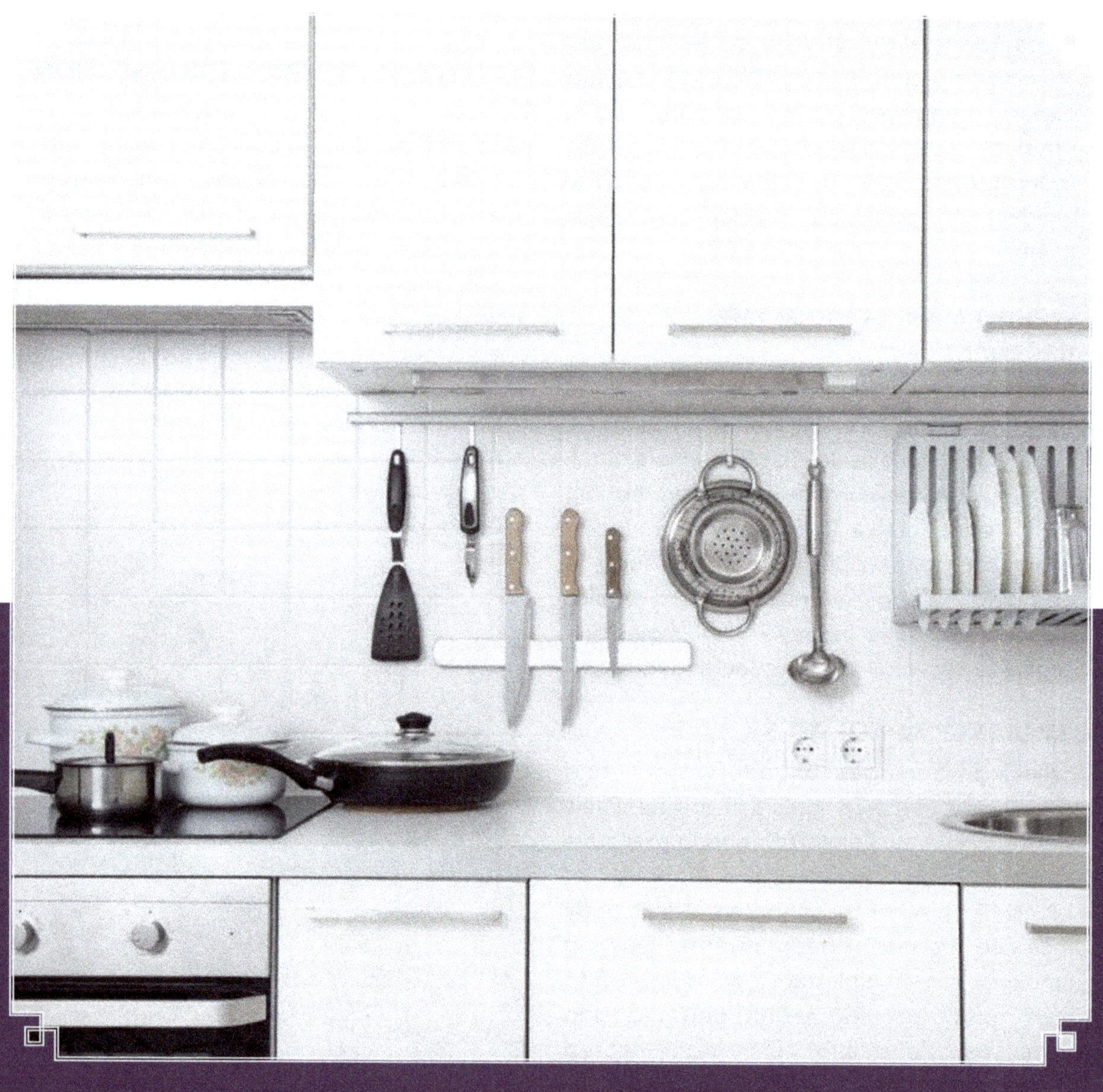

Utensils and Equipment

Creating a low-cholesterol kitchen is a proactive step towards heart-healthy cooking. Equipping your culinary space with the right utensils and equipment can enhance your ability to prepare nutritious and delicious meals. Here are some essential items:

Non-Stick Cookware: Opt for non-stick pans and pots to minimize the need for excessive fats during cooking.

Steamer Basket: A steamer basket is perfect for preparing vegetables, grains, and proteins while retaining their nutrients and flavors.

Baking Sheets and Pans: These are useful for roasting or baking foods without added fats.

Blender or Food Processor: These tools are excellent for creating smoothies, sauces, and dips using heart-healthy ingredients like fruits, vegetables, and nuts.

Citrus Juicer: A manual or electric citrus juicer is handy for adding flavor to dishes without relying on sodium or unhealthy fats.

Quality Knives: Invest in a set of sharp, high-quality knives for efficient and precise food preparation.

Cutting Boards: Choose durable cutting boards for chopping fruits, vegetables, and lean proteins.

Salad Spinner: This helps in washing and drying greens effectively for fresh and crisp salads.

Measuring Cups and Spoons: These ensure accurate portion sizes and control over ingredients.

Herb Grinder or Mortar and Pestle: Enhance flavor without adding excess salt by using freshly ground herbs and spices.

Foods to Focus On

HIGH-FIBER FOODS

Incorporate plenty of whole grains, fruits, vegetables, legumes, and nuts into your diet. These foods are rich in soluble fiber, which helps lower LDL cholesterol levels by binding to cholesterol and aiding in its elimination from the body.

LEAN PROTEINS

Choose lean sources of protein such as skinless poultry, fish (especially fatty fish like salmon and trout), tofu, legumes, and beans. These options provide essential protein without the saturated fat found in red meats.

HEALTHY FATS

Opt for sources of healthy fats, like avocados, nuts, seeds, and olive oil. These fats can help increase HDL cholesterol levels and provide necessary nutrients for overall well-being.

PLANT STEROLS AND STANOLS

Foods fortified with these plant compounds, such as certain margarines, can help reduce LDL cholesterol levels by blocking its absorption.

FATTY ACIDS

Omega-3 fatty acids found in fatty fish, flaxseeds, and walnuts have been shown to support heart health by reducing inflammation and improving cholesterol profiles.

OATS AND BARLEY

These whole grains contain beta-glucans, a type of soluble fiber that can help lower LDL cholesterol levels.

Foods to Avoid

SATURATED FATS

Foods high in saturated fats, such as fatty cuts of red meat, full-fat dairy products, and processed meats like sausages and bacon, can raise LDL cholesterol levels.

TRANS FATS:

Trans fats are often found in processed and fried foods, as well as some margarines and baked goods. They not only raise LDL cholesterol but also lower HDL cholesterol levels.

HIGHLY PROCESSED FOODS

These can contain added sugars, unhealthy fats, and high levels of sodium. Opt for whole, minimally processed foods instead.

EXCESSIVE SODIUM:

High sodium intake can contribute to high blood pressure and negatively impact heart health. Limit processed foods and season meals with herbs and spices instead of salt.

REFINED CARBOHYDRATES

Refined grains like white bread, pastries, and sugary cereals can lead to weight gain and potentially affect cholesterol levels.

FRIED FOODS:

Foods that are deep-fried or heavily battered often contain unhealthy trans fats and can contribute to inflammation and high cholesterol levels.

Cooking Methods

When following a low-cholesterol diet, choosing the right cooking methods can make a significant difference in maintaining your heart health. Opt for methods that require minimal or no added fats and preserve the nutritional integrity of your ingredients. Steaming, baking, grilling, and roasting are excellent options. These methods help retain flavors, textures, and nutrients without the need for excessive oils or butter. By embracing these heart-healthy cooking techniques, you can create flavorful and nourishing meals that contribute to your overall well-being.

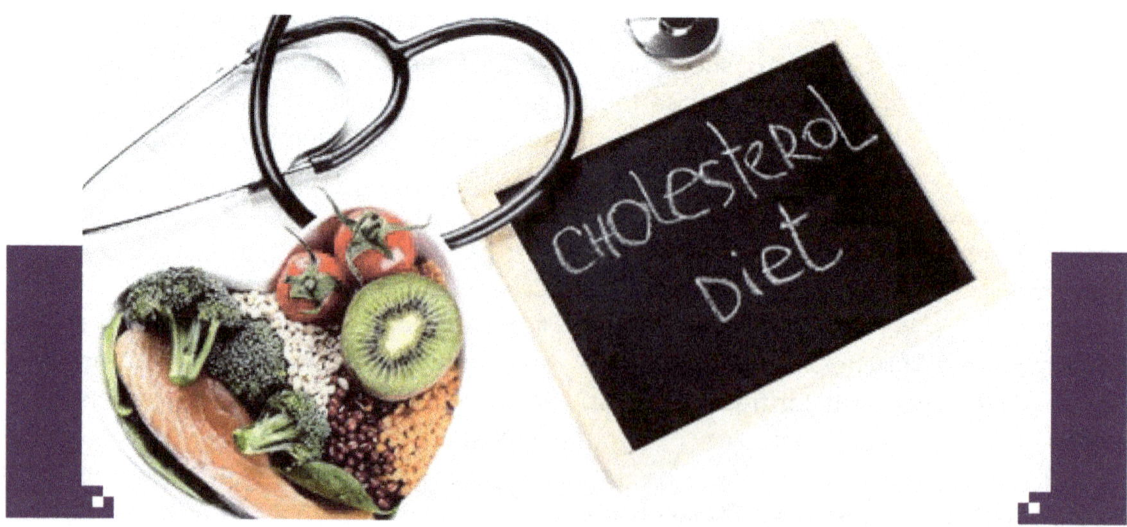

Chapter 3

28-Day Meal Plan

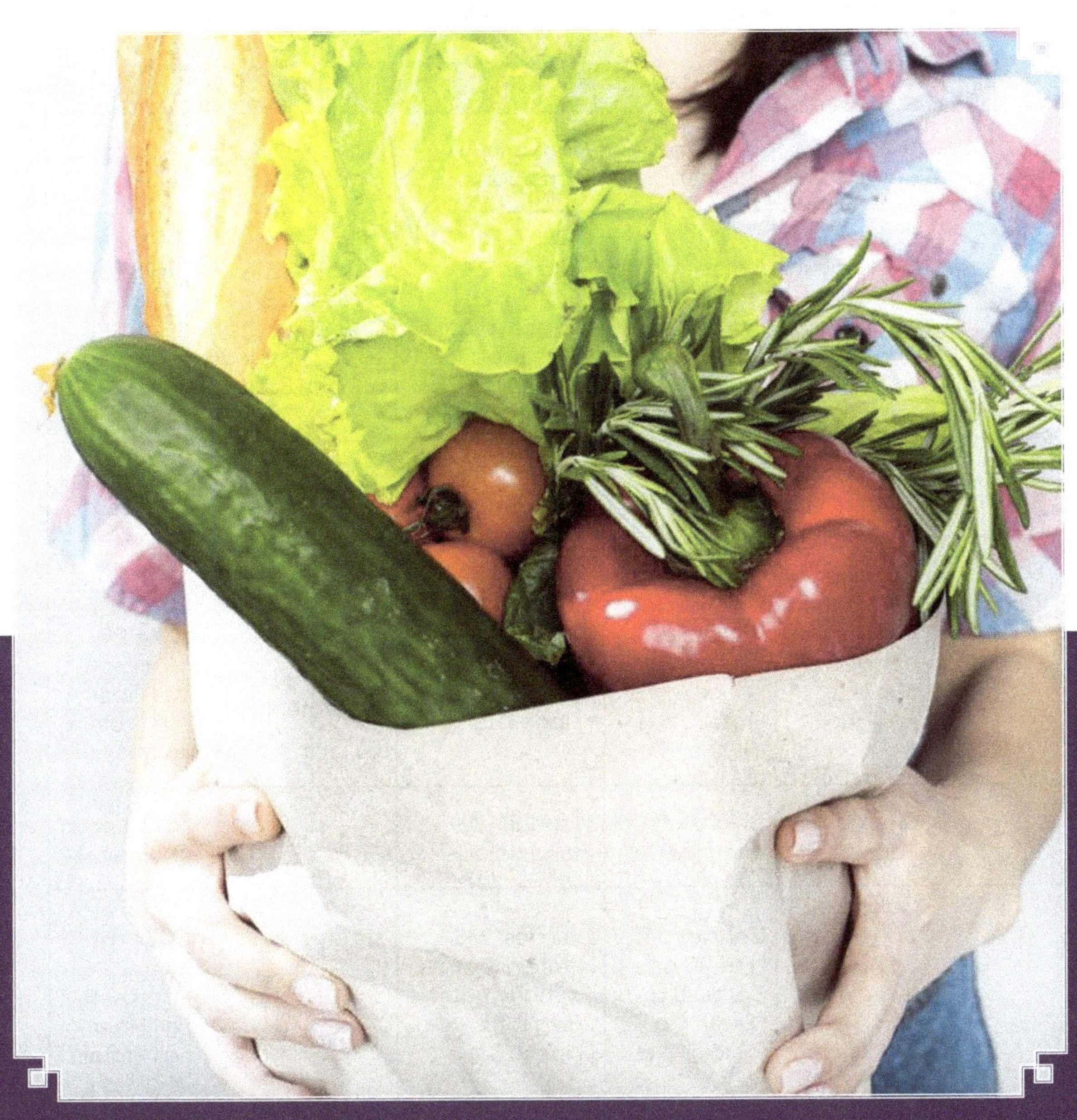

Week 1 Getting Started on Your Low Cholesterol Journey

Welcome to Week 1 of your journey towards better heart health with the Low Cholesterol Cookbook! This week, your focus is on laying a strong foundation for your new dietary habits. Begin by clearing out your kitchen of high cholesterol foods and stocking up on fresh, wholesome options. Plan your meals for the week ahead and make a grocery list to avoid last-minute unhealthy choices.

Start your day with a balanced breakfast that includes fiber-rich foods to keep you full. For lunch and dinner, aim to fill half your plate with colorful vegetables and the other half with lean protein and whole grains. Snack on nuts, seeds, and fruits to curb hunger between meals. Remember, consistency is key, so stick to your plan and stay motivated.

Meal Plan	Breakfast	Snack	Lunch	Dinner	Snack
Day-1	Breakfast Parfaits	Chickpeas Hummus	Mandarin Almond Salad	Mandarin Almond Salad	Chickpeas Hummus
	Calories: 277 | Protein: 5g | Carbohydrates: 60g | Fat: 4g | Fiber: 6 g	Calories: 147 | Fat: 10 g | Carbs: 11 g | Fiber: 4 g | Protein: 6 g	Calories: 235 | Protein: 2g | Carbohydrates: 20.2g | Fat: 16.7g | Fiber: 1.8g	Calories: 235 | Protein: 2g | Carbohydrates: 20.2g | Fat: 16.7g | Fiber: 1.8g	Calories: 147 | Fat: 10 g | Carbs: 11 g | Fiber: 4 g | Protein: 6 g
Day-2	Breakfast Parfaits	Chickpeas Hummus	Mandarin Almond Salad	Cod Satay	Chickpeas Hummus
	Calories: 277 | Protein: 5g | Carbohydrates: 60g | Fat: 4g | Fiber: 6 g	Calories: 147 | Fat: 10 g | Carbs: 11 g | Fiber: 4 g | Protein: 6 g	Calories: 235 | Protein: 2g | Carbohydrates: 20.2g | Fat: 16.7g | Fiber: 1.8g	Calories 255 | Fat: 10g | Carbs:9g | Fiber: 1g | Protein: 33g	Calories: 147 | Fat: 10 g | Carbs: 11 g | Fiber: 4 g | Protein: 6 g
Day-3	Breakfast Parfaits	Chickpeas Hummus	Mandarin Almond Salad	Cod Satay	Chickpeas Hummus
	Calories: 277 | Protein: 5g | Carbohydrates: 60g | Fat: 4g | Fiber: 6 g	Calories: 147 | Fat: 10 g | Carbs: 11 g | Fiber: 4 g | Protein: 6 g	Calories: 235 | Protein: 2g | Carbohydrates: 20.2g | Fat: 16.7g | Fiber: 1.8g	Calories 255 | Fat: 10g | Carbs:9g | Fiber: 1g | Protein: 33g	Calories: 147 | Fat: 10 g | Carbs: 11 g | Fiber: 4 g | Protein: 6 g

Day-4	Breakfast Parfaits	Chickpeas Hummus	Mandarin Almond Salad	Cod Satay	Chickpeas Hummus
	Calories: 277 | Protein: 5g | Carbohydrates: 60g | Fat: 4g | Fiber: 6 g	Calories: 147 | Fat: 10 g | Carbs: 11 g | Fiber: 4 g | Protein: 6 g	Calories: 235 | Protein: 2g | Carbohydrates: 20.2g | Fat: 16.7g | Fiber: 1.8g	Calories 255 | Fat: 10g | Carbs:9g | Fiber: 1g | Protein: 33g	Calories: 147 | Fat: 10 g | Carbs: 11 g | Fiber: 4 g | Protein: 6 g
Day-5	Creamy Oats Banana Porridge	Roasted Red Pepper Hummus	Mandarin Almond Salad	Cod Satay	Roasted Red Pepper Hummus
	Calories: 323 | Fat:16.6 g | Carbohydrates: 37.6 g | Protein: 9.6 g	Calories: 130 | Total fat: 8g | Total Carbohydrates: 11g | Fiber: 2g |Protein: 4g	Calories: 235 | Protein: 2g | Carbohydrates: 20.2g | Fat: 16.7g | Fiber: 1.8g	Calories 255 | Fat: 10g | Carbs:9g | Fiber: 1g | Protein: 33g	Calories: 130 | Total fat: 8g | Total Carbohydrates: 11g | Fiber: 2g |Protein: 4g

Shopping List for Week 1

PROTEINS:

- 4 (6-ounce) cod fillets
- 1 (15 ounces) can chickpeas, drained and rinsed
- 1 (15-ounce) can low-sodium chickpeas, drained and rinsed

VEGETABLES:

- 6 thinly sliced green onions
- 1 small onion, diced
- 2 cloves garlic, minced
- 1 tomato, chopped

FRUITS:

- 1 cup of fresh/frozen raspberries
- 2 cups of pineapple chunks
- 1 cup of sliced ripe banana
- ½ banana, mashed
- 2 (11 ounces) cans of mandarin oranges, drained

MISCELLANEOUS:

- 1/4 cup of sliced almonds
- 1/2 cup of chopped dates or raisins
- 1/4 cup sliced almonds
- 1/2 cup olive oil
- 1/4 cup red wine vinegar
- 1 tablespoon white sugar
- 1 tablespoon packed brown sugar
- 2 tablespoons low-sodium vegetable broth
- 2 teaspoons low-sodium soy sauce
- 3 tablespoons sesame tahini
- 3 ounces jarred roasted red bell peppers, drained
- 3 tablespoons lemon juice
- 1 garlic clove, peeled
- 3 tablespoons extra-virgin olive oil
- Fresh herbs, chopped, for garnish (optional)

NUTS:

- 1/4 cup of sliced almonds

Week 2 Exploring Flavorful Choices

As you enter Week 2, you're already on your way to healthier eating habits. This week, let's focus on adding exciting flavors to your meals without compromising on health. Experiment with herbs, spices, and different cooking techniques to make your dishes more appealing. Replace saturated fats with healthier options like olive oil or avocado.

Get creative with your breakfast by trying out different combinations of grains, fruits, and nuts. For lunch, opt for colorful salads with a variety of veggies and a lean protein source. At dinner, explore plant-based proteins like beans and lentils. Keep your taste buds engaged with satisfying snacks that combine sweet, savory, and crunchy elements. Remember, a flavorful diet is a sustainable one.

Meal Plan	Breakfast	Snack	Lunch	Dinner	Snack
Day-1	Tomato Basil Bruschetta	Turkey Cocktail Meatballs	Mexican Bean Salad	Mexican Bean Salad	Turkey Cocktail Meatballs
	Calories: 142	Protein: 5g	Carbohydrates: 26g	Fat: 2g |Fiber: 2 g	Calories: 100	Protein: 10g	Carbohydrates: 9g	Fat: 2g	Fiber: 0g	Calories: 172	Protein: 9g	Carbohydrates: 29g	Fat: 3g	Fiber: 7g	Calories: 172	Protein: 9g	Carbohydrates: 29g	Fat: 3g	Fiber: 7g	Calories: 100	Protein: 10g	Carbohydrates: 9g	Fat: 2g	Fiber: 0g
Day-2	Tomato Basil Bruschetta	Turkey Cocktail Meatballs	Mexican Bean Salad	Mexican Bean Salad	Turkey Cocktail Meatballs
	Calories: 142	Protein: 5g	Carbohydrates: 26g	Fat: 2g |Fiber: 2 g	Calories: 100	Protein: 10g	Carbohydrates: 9g	Fat: 2g	Fiber: 0g	Calories: 172	Protein: 9g	Carbohydrates: 29g	Fat: 3g	Fiber: 7g	Calories: 172	Protein: 9g	Carbohydrates: 29g	Fat: 3g	Fiber: 7g	Calories: 100	Protein: 10g	Carbohydrates: 9g	Fat: 2g	Fiber: 0g
Day-3	Tomato Basil Bruschetta	Turkey Cocktail Meatballs	Mexican Bean Salad	Mexican Bean Salad	Turkey Cocktail Meatballs
	Calories: 142	Protein: 5g	Carbohydrates: 26g	Fat: 2g |Fiber: 2 g	Calories: 100	Protein: 10g	Carbohydrates: 9g	Fat: 2g	Fiber: 0g	Calories: 172	Protein: 9g	Carbohydrates: 29g	Fat: 3g	Fiber: 7g	Calories: 172	Protein: 9g	Carbohydrates: 29g	Fat: 3g	Fiber: 7g	Calories: 100	Protein: 10g	Carbohydrates: 9g	Fat: 2g	Fiber: 0g

Day-4	Tomato Basil Bruschetta	Turkey Cocktail Meatballs	Mexican Bean Salad	Mexican Bean Salad	Turkey Cocktail Meatballs
	Calories: 142 | Protein: 5g | Carbohydrates: 26g | Fat: 2g |Fiber: 2 g	Calories: 100 | Protein: 10g | Carbohydrates: 9g | Fat: 2g | Fiber: 0g	Calories: 172 | Protein: 9g | Carbohydrates: 29g | Fat: 3g | Fiber: 7g	Calories: 172 | Protein: 9g | Carbohydrates: 29g | Fat: 3g | Fiber: 7g	Calories: 100 | Protein: 10g | Carbohydrates: 9g | Fat: 2g | Fiber: 0g
Day-5	Tomato Basil Bruschetta	Turkey Cocktail Meatballs	Olive Turkey Patties	Olive Turkey Patties	Turkey Cocktail Meatballs
	Calories: 142 | Protein: 5g | Carbdrates: 26g | Fat: 2g |Fiber: 2 g	Calories: 100 | Protein: 10g | Carbohydrates: 9g | Fat: 2g | Fiber: 0g	Calories: 366 | Total Fat: 15g | Total Carbs: 35g | Fiber: 6g | Protein: 24g	Calories: 366 | Total Fat: 15g | Total Carbs: 35g | Fiber: 6g | Protein: 24g	Calories: 100 | Protein: 10g | Carbohydrates: 9g | Fat: 2g | Fiber: 0g

Shopping List for Week 2

PROTEINS:

- 2 cups cooked kidney beans
- 2 cups cooked garbanzo beans
- 1 lb. lean ground turkey
- 1-pound ground turkey breast

VEGETABLES:

- 3 diced tomatoes
- 1/2 cup diced fennel
- 3/4 cup cucumber, peeled & chopped
- 4 cups lettuce, shredded
- 2 tablespoons diced onion
- ¼ cup sliced black olives, chopped
- ¼ cup white onion, finely chopped
- ¼ cup parsley, finely chopped
- 1 tbsp garlic, minced
- 6 beefsteak tomato slices
- ¼ cup chopped onion
- ¼ cup chopped green bell pepper

HERBS AND SPICES:

- 2 tablespoons chopped basil
- 1 tablespoon chopped parsley
- 2 teaspoons balsamic vinegar
- 1/2 teaspoon black pepper
- 1/4 teaspoon minced garlic
- 1/2 teaspoon cumin
- 1/2 teaspoon ground ginger
- 1/4 teaspoon onion powder

CONDIMENTS AND SAUCES:

- 2 teaspoons Dijon mustard
- 1 1/4 cups unsweetened pineapple juice
- 6 tablespoons Dijon mustard, divided
- 1 tablespoon honey
- 1 tablespoon cornstarch

BAKERY:

- 1/2 whole-grain baguette, six 1/2-inch-thick diagonal slices
- 6 whole-wheat hamburger buns

FRUITS:

- 1/2 cup avocado, mashed
- 1 ripe avocado, peeled, pitted, and sliced

DAIRY:

- 1/2 cup plain fat-free yogurt
- 4 ounces part-skim shredded mozzarella
- 1/4 cup egg substitute

OTHER:

- ½ cup rolled oats
- Aluminum foil

Week 3 Mindful Eating and Portion Awareness

Welcome to Week 3, where the focus shifts to mindful eating and portion control. Take time to savor each bite, and pay attention to your body's hunger and fullness cues. Avoid distractions during meals and eat slowly. This week, practice listening to your body and enjoying your food without overindulging.

Begin your day with a nourishing breakfast that includes a mix of nutrients to keep you energized. Opt for balanced lunches and dinners that feature a variety of colorful vegetables, lean proteins, and whole grains. Keep healthy snacks on hand to avoid reaching for unhealthy choices when hunger strikes. By eating mindfully and being aware of portion sizes, you'll build a healthier relationship with food

Meal Plan	Breakfast	Snack	Lunch	Dinner	Snack
Day-1	Overnight Peach Oatmeal	Fat-Free Potato Chips	Bavarian Beef	Roasted Vegetable Stuffed Pizza	Fat-Free Potato Chips
	Calories: 163 kcal | Protein: 5g | Carbohydrates: 31g | Fat: 2g |Fiber: 4 g	Calories: 129 | Protein: 3g | Carbohydrates: 29g | Fat: 0g | Fiber: 3g	Calories: 218 kcal | Protein: 24g | Carbohydrates: 14g | Fat: 7g | Fiber: 1 g	Calories: 393 kcal | Protein: 15g | Carbohydrates: 62g | Fat: 11g | Fiber: 8 g	Calories: 129 | Protein: 3g | Carbohydrates: 29g | Fat: 0g | Fiber: 3g
Day-2	Overnight Peach Oatmeal	Fat-Free Potato Chips	Bavarian Beef	Roasted Vegetable Stuffed Pizza	Fat-Free Potato Chips
	Calories: 163 kcal | Protein: 5g | Carbohydrates: 31g | Fat: 2g |Fiber: 4 g	Calories: 129 | Protein: 3g | Carbohydrates: 29g | Fat: 0g | Fiber: 3g	Calories: 218 kcal | Protein: 24g | Carbohydrates: 14g | Fat: 7g | Fiber: 1 g	Calories: 393 kcal | Protein: 15g | Carbohydrates: 62g | Fat: 11g | Fiber: 8 g	Calories: 129 | Protein: 3g | Carbohydrates: 29g | Fat: 0g | Fiber: 3g
Day-3	Overnight Peach Oatmeal	Fat-Free Potato Chips	Bavarian Beef	Roasted Vegetable Stuffed Pizza	Fat-Free Potato Chips
	Calories: 163 kcal | Protein: 5g | Carbohydrates: 31g | Fat: 2g |Fiber: 4 g	Calories: 129 | Protein: 3g | Carbohydrates: 29g | Fat: 0g | Fiber: 3g	Calories: 218 kcal | Protein: 24g | Carbohydrates: 14g | Fat: 7g | Fiber: 1 g	Calories: 393 kcal | Protein: 15g | Carbohydrates: 62g | Fat: 11g | Fiber: 8 g	Calories: 129 | Protein: 3g | Carbohydrates: 29g | Fat: 0g | Fiber: 3g

Day-4	Overnight Peach Oatmeal	Fat-Free Potato Chips	Bavarian Beef	Roasted Vegetable Stuffed Pizza	Fat-Free Potato Chips
	Calories: 163 kcal | Protein: 5g | Carbohydrates: 31g | Fat: 2g |Fiber: 4 g	Calories: 129 | Protein: 3g | Carbohydrates: 29g | Fat: 0g | Fiber: 3g	Calories: 218 kcal | Protein: 24g | Carbohydrates: 14g | Fat: 7g | Fiber: 1 g	Calories: 393 kcal | Protein: 15g | Carbohydrates: 62g | Fat: 11g | Fiber: 8 g	Calories: 129 | Protein: 3g | Carbohydrates: 29g | Fat: 0g | Fiber: 3g
Day-5	Overnight Peach Oatmeal	Cherry Tomato Bruschetta	Bavarian Beef	Roasted Vegetable Stuffed Pizza	Cherry Tomato Bruschetta
	Calories: 163 kcal | Protein: 5g | Carbohydrates: 31g | Fat: 2g |Fiber: 4 g	Calories: 100 | Total fat: 6g | Total Carbohydrates: 10g | Fiber: 2g | Protein: 4g	Calories: 218 kcal | Protein: 24g | Carbohydrates: 14g | Fat: 7g | Fiber: 1 g	Calories: 393 kcal | Protein: 15g | Carbohydrates: 62g | Fat: 11g | Fiber: 8 g	Calories: 100 | Total fat: 6g | Total Carbohydrates: 10g | Fiber: 2g | Protein: 4g

Shopping List for Week 3

PROTEINS:

- 1 1/4 lb. of lean beef/stew meat, cut into 1-inch pieces

VEGETABLES:

- 2 medium peaches, sliced / 3 cups unsweetened frozen sliced peaches, thawed
- 1/2 small head of red cabbage, cut into 4 wedges
- 3 cups mushrooms, quartered
- 2 cups zucchini, sliced
- 1 cup onion, sliced
- 1 cup red bell pepper, sliced
- 1 cup green bell pepper, sliced
- 4 medium potatoes
- 8 ounces assorted cherry tomatoes, halved
- Fresh herbs, chopped (such as basil, parsley, tarragon, dill)

FRUITS:

- 2 medium peaches, sliced / 3 cups unsweetened frozen sliced peaches, thawed

MISCELLANEOUS:

- 1 cup steel-cut oats
- 1/4 teaspoon salt
- 1/4 teaspoon vanilla/almond extract
- 3 tablespoons brown sugar
- 1 cup vanilla soy milk/vanilla almond milk
- 1 tbsp vegetable oil
- 1/8 tsp black pepper
- 1/4 cup crushed gingersnaps
- 1 large thinly sliced onion
- 1 1/2 cups water
- 3/4 tsp caraway seeds
- 1/2 tsp salt
- 1/4 cup white vinegar
- 1 bay leaf
- 1 tbsp sugar
- 1 cup water
- 4 teaspoons olive oil
- 1 1/2 cups bread flour
- 1 1/2 cups whole wheat flour
- 1 1/2 teaspoons yeast

- Your choice of spices or herbs
- ⅓ cup fresh herbs, chopped (such as basil, parsley, tarragon, dill)
- 1 tablespoon extra-virgin olive oil
- ¼ teaspoon kosher salt
- ⅛ teaspoon freshly ground black pepper
- ¼ cup ricotta cheese

NUTS:
- Optional toppings: sliced almonds

DAIRY:
- 3 ounces part-skim mozzarella, shredded

BAKERY:
- 4 slices whole-wheat bread, toasted

Week 4 Sustaining Progress and Looking Ahead

Congratulations, you've reached Week 4 – the final week of your journey with the Low Cholesterol Cookbook! This week is all about maintaining the progress you've made and setting your sights on the future. Reflect on the positive changes you've incorporated into your diet and how they've made you feel.

Continue to choose nutrient-dense foods for your meals, emphasizing variety and balance. Start your day with a wholesome breakfast, and continue to enjoy colorful salads and well-rounded dinners. Snack smartly and stay hydrated throughout the day. As you complete this four-week plan, celebrate your accomplishments and consider the next steps in your health journey. Remember, this is just the beginning of a lifelong commitment to better well-being. Keep up the great work!

Meal Plan	Breakfast	Snack	Lunch	Dinner	Snack
Day-1	Blueberry Muffins	Easy Pizza	Shrimp Pasta Primavera	Shrimp Pasta Primavera	Easy Pizza
	Calories: 204 | Protein: 5.8g | Carbohydrates: 14.9g | Fat: 14.6g | Fiber: 2.9g	Calories: 247 kcal | Protein: 4g | Carbohydrates: 32g | Fat: 12g |Fiber: 1 g	Total Calories: 369 | Total Fat: 7g Total Carbohydrate: 43g | Fiber: 9g | Protein: 30g	Total Calories: 369 | Total Fat: 7g Total Carbohydrate: 43g | Fiber: 9g | Protein: 30g	Calories: 247 kcal | Protein: 4g | Carbohydrates: 32g | Fat: 12g |Fiber: 1 g
Day-2	Blueberry Muffins	Easy Pizza	Shrimp Pasta Primavera	Lentil Pilaf	Easy Pizza
	Calories: 204 | Protein: 5.8g | Carbohydrates: 14.9g | Fat: 14.6g | Fiber: 2.9g	Calories: 247 kcal | Protein: 4g | Carbohydrates: 32g | Fat: 12g |Fiber: 1 g	Total Calories: 369 | Total Fat: 7g Total Carbohydrate: 43g | Fiber: 9g | Protein: 30g	Calories: 348 | Fat: 6g | Carbs: 59g | Dietary Fiber: 11g | Protein: 19g	Calories: 247 kcal | Protein: 4g | Carbohydrates: 32g | Fat: 12g |Fiber: 1 g

Day-3	Blueberry Muffins	Easy Pizza	Shrimp Pasta Primavera	Lentil Pilaf	Easy Pizza
	Calories: 204	Protein: 5.8g	Carbohydrates: 14.9g	Fat: 14.6g	Fiber: 2.9g	Calories: 247 kcal	Protein: 4g	Carbohydrates: 32g	Fat: 12g |Fiber: 1 g	Total Calories: 369	Total Fat: 7g Total Carbohydrate: 43g	Fiber: 9g	Protein: 30g	Calories: 348	Fat: 6g	Carbs: 59g	Dietary Fiber: 11g	Protein: 19g	Calories: 247 kcal	Protein: 4g	Carbohydrates: 32g	Fat: 12g |Fiber: 1 g
Day-4	Blueberry Muffins	Easy Pizza	Shrimp Pasta Primavera	Lentil Pilaf	Easy Pizza
	Calories: 204	Protein: 5.8g	Carbohydrates: 14.9g	Fat: 14.6g	Fiber: 2.9g	Calories: 247 kcal	Protein: 4g	Carbohydrates: 32g	Fat: 12g |Fiber: 1 g	Total Calories: 369	Total Fat: 7g Total Carbohydrate: 43g	Fiber: 9g	Protein: 30g	Calories: 348	Fat: 6g	Carbs: 59g	Dietary Fiber: 11g	Protein: 19g	Calories: 247 kcal	Protein: 4g	Carbohydrates: 32g	Fat: 12g |Fiber: 1 g
Day-5	Blueberry Muffins	Easy Pizza	Shrimp Pasta Primavera	Lentil Pilaf	Easy Pizza
	Calories: 204	Protein: 5.8g	Carbohydrates: 14.9g	Fat: 14.6g	Fiber: 2.9g	Calories: 247 kcal	Protein: 4g	Carbohydrates: 32g	Fat: 12g |Fiber: 1 g	Total Calories: 369	Total Fat: 7g Total Carbohydrate: 43g	Fiber: 9g	Protein: 30g	Calories: 348	Fat: 6g	Carbs: 59g	Dietary Fiber: 11g	Protein: 19g	Calories: 247 kcal	Protein: 4g	Carbohydrates: 32g	Fat: 12g |Fiber: 1 g

Shopping List for Week 4

BAKING:

- ¼ cup coconut flour
- 1 ¾ cups almond flour
- ¼ teaspoon baking soda

FRUITS:

- 1 cup blueberries
- zest and juice of 1 lemon

DAIRY:

- ½ cup reduced-fat milk

SPICES AND SEASONINGS:

- ¼ teaspoon salt
- ¾ teaspoon kosher or sea salt

VEGETABLES:

- 1 small head broccoli, chopped
- 1 red bell pepper, seeded and chopped

LEGUMES:

- 1¼ cup Puy lentils

LIQUIDS:

- 2 tablespoons chopped fresh basil
- ½ cup unsalted vegetable, chicken, or fish stock

NUTS:

- 1/2 cup dry-roasted peanuts, chopped

MISCELLANEOUS:

- 12 ounces whole-grain spaghetti
- 1 cup frozen green peas

Chapter 4

Breakfast and Smoothies

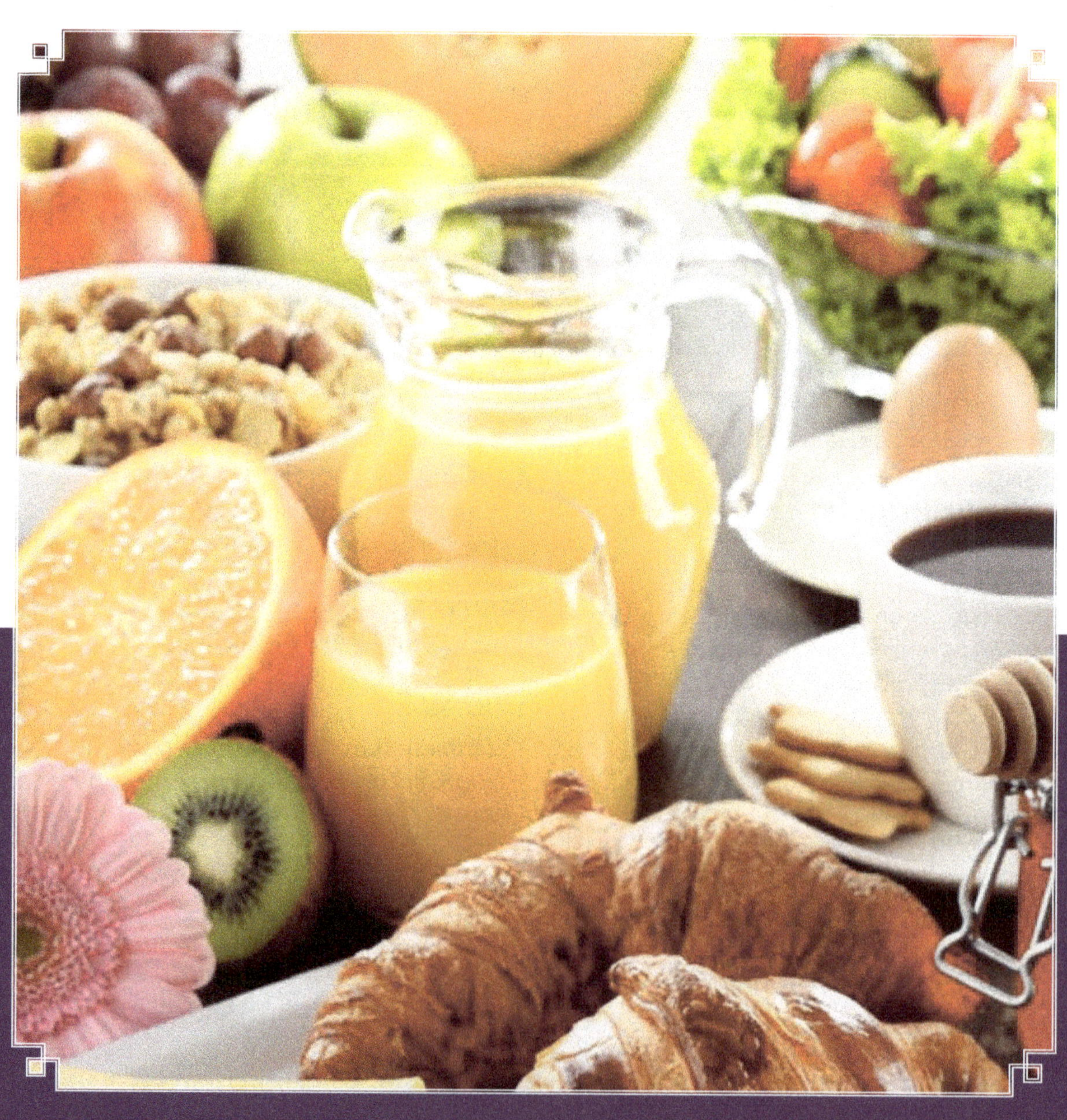

Berry Smoothie Bowl

**Prep time: 5 minutes | Cook time: 5 minutes |
Serves 2**

- 1 cup of fat-free milk
- 1 cup of frozen unsweetened strawberries
- 1/2 cup of frozen unsweetened raspberries
- 3 tablespoons of sugar
- 1 cup of ice cubes
- optional: sliced fresh strawberries, chia seeds, unsweetened shredded coconut, fresh raspberries, fresh pumpkin seeds, and sliced almonds

1. Combine the milk, berries, and sugar in a blender; cover and mix until smooth.
2. Cover and process until smooth, adding ice cubes as needed.
3. To serve, divide the mixture into two serving dishes.
4. Optional toppings may be added as desired.

PER SERVING

Calories: 155 kcal | Protein: 5g | Carbohydrates: 35g | Fat: 0g | Cholesterol: 2 mg | Fiber: 2g

Breakfast Parfaits

**Prep time: 10 minutes | Cook time: 10 minutes |
Serves 4**

- 1 cup of fresh/frozen raspberries
- 2 cups of pineapple chunks
- 1 cup of vanilla yogurt
- 1/2 cup of chopped dates or raisins
- 1/4 cup of sliced almonds
- 1 cup of sliced ripe banana

1. Layer the yogurt, dates, raspberries, pineapple, and banana in 4 parfait glasses or serving plates.
2. Almonds are sprinkled on top.
3. Serve right away.

PER SERVING

Calories: 277 kcal | Protein: 5g | Carbohydrates: 60g | Fat: 4g | Cholesterol: 3mg | Fiber: 6 g

Tomato Basil Bruschetta

**Prep time: 5 minutes | Cook time: 5 minutes |
Serves 6**

- 2 tablespoons of chopped basil
- 1/2 whole-grain baguette, six 1/2-inch-thick diagonal slices
- 1 tablespoon of chopped parsley
- 3 diced tomatoes,
- 2 minced cloves garlic,
- 1 teaspoon of olive oil
- 1/2 cup of diced fennel
- 1 teaspoon of black pepper
- 2 teaspoons of balsamic vinegar

1. Preheat the oven to 400 degrees Fahrenheit.
2. Baguette pieces should be gently toasted.
3. Combine all the remaining in a large mixing bowl.
4. Distribute the mixture equally over the toasted bread.
5. Serve right away.

PER SERVING

Calories: 142 kcal | Protein: 5g | Carbohydrates: 26g | Fat: 2g | Cholesterol: 0mg | Fiber: 2 g

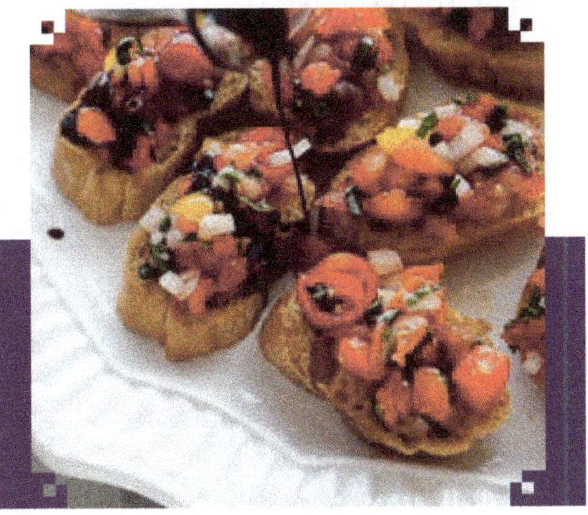

Creamy Oats Banana Porridge

Prep time: 10 minutes | Cook time: 5 minutes | Serves 1

- ¼ cup steel-cut oats
- 1 tbsp peanut butter
- ½ tsp vanilla
- ½ tbsp chia seeds
- ½ banana, mashed
- ½ cup unsweetened almond milk
- 1 cup water

1. Add oats and water to a saucepan and bring to boil.
2. Once oats begin to thicken, add vanilla, chia seeds, mashed banana, and almond milk and cook over low heat for 5 minutes. Stir constantly.
3. Top with peanut butter and serve.

PER SERVING

Calories: 323 | Fat:16.6 g | Carbohydrates: 37.6 g | Sugar: 8.4 g | Protein: 9.6 g | Cholesterol: 0 mg

Overnight Peach Oatmeal

Prep time: 10 minutes | Cook time: 7 hours 10 minutes | Serves 6

- 1 cup of steel-cut oats
- 1/4 teaspoon of salt
- 4 cups of water
- 1/4 teaspoon of vanilla/ almond extract
- 3 tablespoons of brown sugar
- 1 cup of vanilla soy milk/ vanilla almond milk
- optional toppings: brown sugar, cinnamon, sliced almonds, and additional peaches
- 2 medium peaches; sliced/ 3 cups of unsweetened frozen sliced peaches, thawed

1. Mix the first 6 in a well-greased 3-quart slow cooker.
2. Cook on low for 7-8 hours, covered until oats are soft.
3. Just before serving, add the peaches.
4. Pressure cooker option: Reduce the amount of water to 3 cups.
5. Pour into a 6-quart electric pressure cooker that has been sprayed with cooking spray.
6. Add the soy milk, oats, salt, brown sugar, and vanilla.
7. Close the pressure-release valve and lock the lid.
8. Adjust to high pressure and cook for 4 minutes.

PER SERVING

Calories: 163 kcal | Protein: 5g | Carbohydrates: 31g | Fat: 2g | Cholesterol: 0mg | Fiber: 4 g

Mango Oat Smoothie

Prep time: 5 minutes | Cook time: 5 minutes | Serves 3

- 1/4 cup of old-fashioned oats
- 2 cups of frozen mango
- 1 banana: (frozen is better)
- 2 cups of oat milk /other plant-based milk /skim milk
- 1/4 lemon/orange (juiced)
- 1 tablespoon of ground flax seed

1. In a blender, combine all of the .
2. Blend until completely smooth.
3. Pour into three glasses and enjoy!

PER SERVING

Calories: 201 kcal | Protein: 8g | Carbohydrates: 39g | Fat: 3g | Cholesterol: 3mg | Fiber: 4g

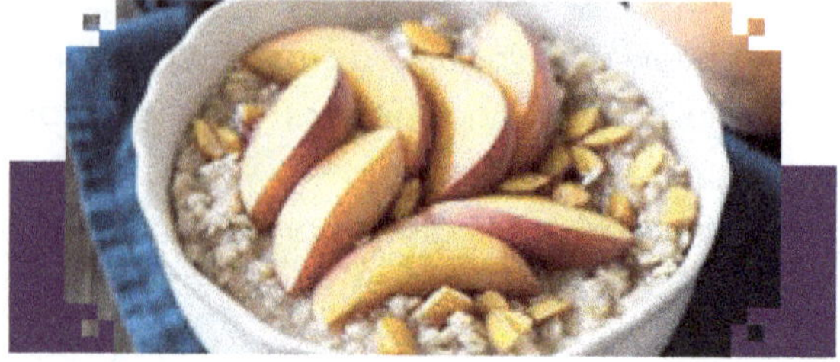

Easy Egg Breakfast Muffins

Prep time: 10 minutes | Cook time: 25 minutes | Serves 12

- 2 ½ cups egg whites
- 1 tbsp fresh parsley, chopped
- ¼ cup cheddar cheese, shredded
- ½ cup cherry tomatoes, quartered
- 1 cup fresh baby spinach, chopped
- Pepper
- Salt

1. Preheat the oven to 350 F/ 180 C.
2. Whisk together egg whites, cheese, pepper, and salt in a bowl.
3. Add parsley, tomatoes, and spinach and stir until well mixed.
4. Pour egg mixture into the greased muffin pan and bake in preheated oven for 25 minutes.
5. Serve and enjoy.

PER SERVING

Calories: 30 | Fat:0.2 g | Carbohydrates: 0.8 g | Sugar: 0.6 g | Protein: 5.8 g | Cholesterol: 0 mg

Protein Packed Quinoa

Prep time: 10 minutes | Cook time: 15 minutes | Serves 2

- ½ cup quinoa, uncooked
- 1 tbsp peanut butter
- 1 ½ tbsp honey
- ½ tsp cinnamon
- 1 ¼ cup unsweetened almond milk

1. Add quinoa and almond milk to a saucepan and bring to a boil.
2. Turn heat to low and simmer for 15 minutes or until quinoa is cooked.
3. Add honey and peanut butter and stir well. Turn off the heat.
4. Top with chopped nuts and serve.

PER SERVING

Calories: 271 | Fat:9.3 g | Carbohydrates: 40.6 g | Sugar: 9.3 g | Protein: 8.4 g | Cholesterol: 0 mg

Blueberry Muffins

Prep time: 15 minutes | Cook time: 1 hour | Serves 12

- ¼ cup of coconut flour
- 1 ¾ cups of almond flour
- ¼ teaspoon of baking soda
- 1 tablespoon of baking powder
- 1 cup of blueberries
- 1 ½ teaspoon of vanilla extract
- ¼ teaspoon of salt
- ½ cup of reduced-fat milk
- 3 large eggs
- ¼ cup of avocado oil

1. Preheat an oven to 350 degrees Fahrenheit.
2. Using cooking spray, generously coat a muffin tray.
3. Sift together coconut flour, baking soda, almond flour, baking powder, and salt in a large mixing bowl.
4. Toss in the blueberries to coat.
5. Whisk the brown sugar, eggs, oil, milk, and vanilla extract in a medium mixing bowl.

PER SERVING

Calories: 204 kcal | Protein: 5.8g | Carbohydrates: 14.9g | Fat: 14.6g | Cholesterol: 47.3mg | Fiber: 2.9g

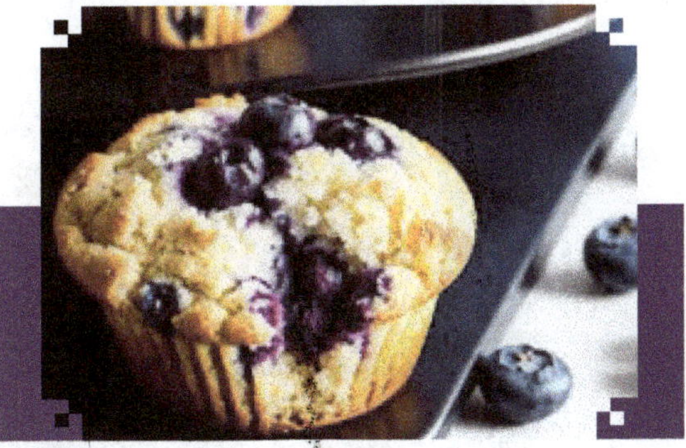

Chapter 5

Snacks and Sides

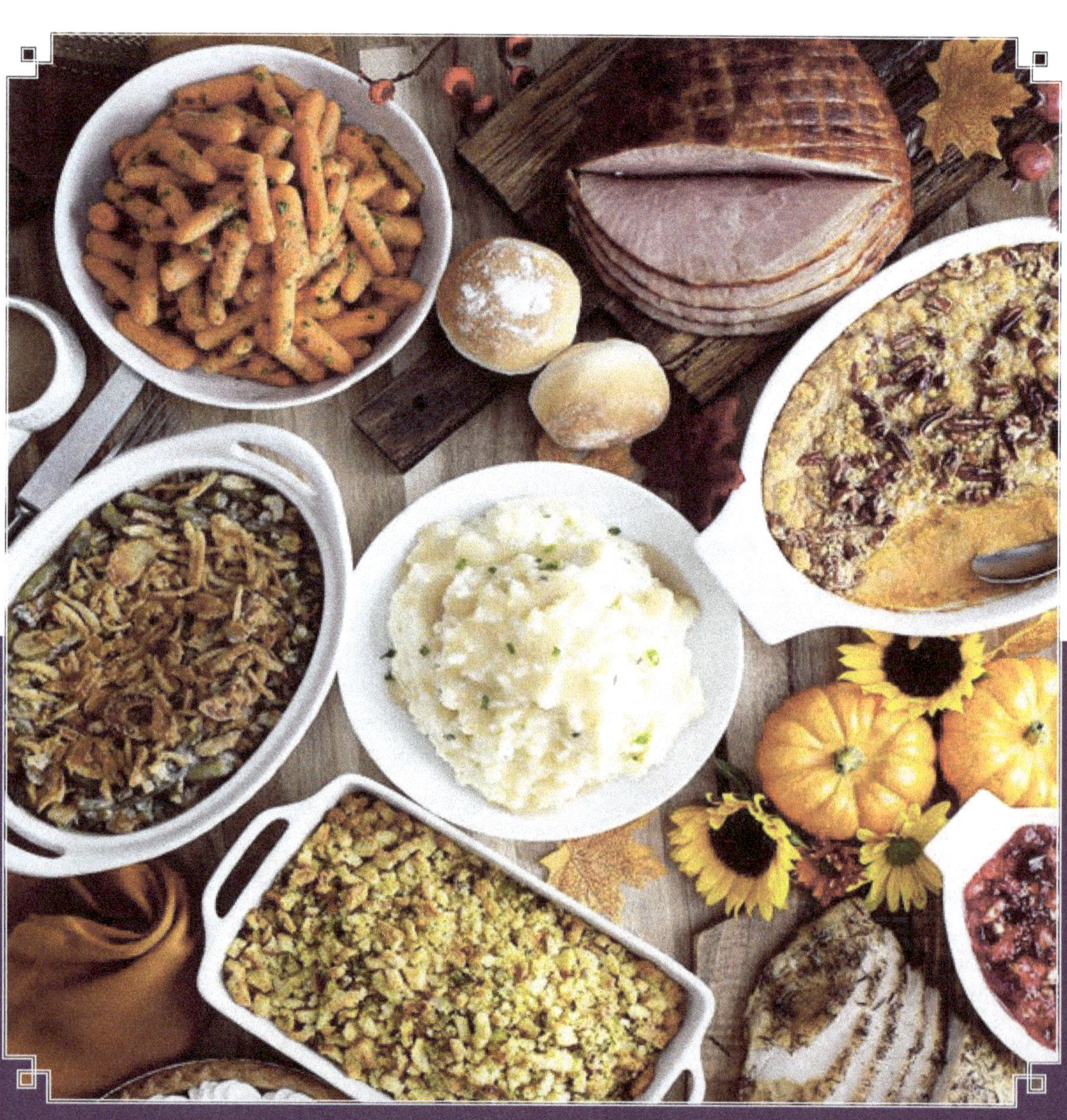

Sour Cream Green Beans

Prep time: 10 minutes | Cook time: 4 hours | Serves 8

- 15 ounces green beans
- 14 ounces corn
- 4 ounces mushrooms, sliced
- 11 ounces cream of mushroom soup, low-fat and sodium-free
- ½ cup low-fat sour cream
- ½ cup almonds, chopped
- ½ cup low-fat Cheddar cheese, shredded

1. In your slow cooker, mix the green beans with the corn, mushrooms soup, mushrooms, almonds, cheese and sour cream, toss
2. cover and cook on low for 4 hours.
3. Stir one more time, divide between plates and serve as a side dish.

PER SERVING

Calories: 360 | Fat: 12.7g | Sodium: 220mg | Carbs: 58.3g | Fiber: 10g | Sugar: 10.3g | Protein: 14g

Fat-Free Potato Chips

Prep time: 10 minutes | Cook time: 25 minutes | Serves 8

- 4 medium potatoes
- your choice of spices or herbs

1. Peel the potatoes before slicing.
2. If desired, season with your favorite spices or herbs.
3. Place the sliced potatoes in a single layer on a microwave bacon tray if you have one.
4. Cover with a spherical, hefty plastic cover that can be microwaved.
5. Place potatoes between two microwave-safe plates if you don't have a bacon tray.
6. Microwave for 7 to 8 minutes on high (full power).
7. Depending on the wattage of your microwave, the cooking time may vary slightly.
8. The sliced potatoes do not need to be turned over.
9. By the time you finish, the plates will be hot.

PER SERVING

Calories: 129 kcal | Protein: 3g | Carbohydrates: 29g | Fat: 0g | Cholesterol: 0mg | Fiber: 3g

Chickpeas Hummus

Prep time: 10 minutes | Cook time: 0 minutes | Serves 8

- 1 (15 ounces) can chickpeas, drained and rinsed
- 3 tablespoons sesame tahini
- 2 tablespoons olive oil
- 3 garlic cloves, chopped
- 1 lemon juice
- Salt and black pepper, to taste

1. In a food processor or blender, combine all the ingredients: until smooth but thick.
2. Add water, if necessary, to produce smoother hummus.
3. Store covered for up 5 days.

PER SERVING

Calories: 147 | Fat: 10 g | Sodium: 64 mg | Carbs: 11 g | Fiber: 4 g | Sugar: 0 g | Protein: 6 g

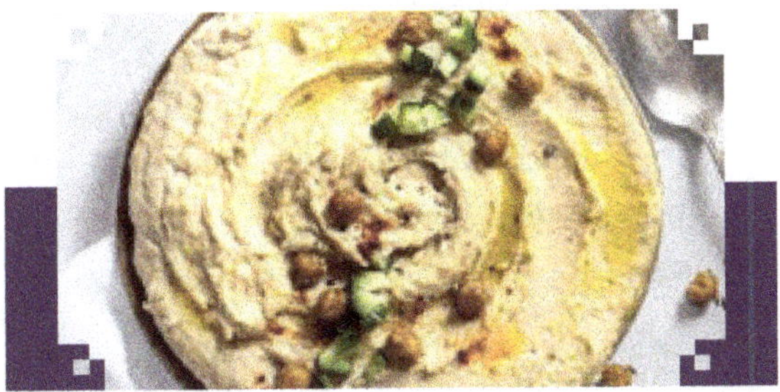

Edamame and Avocado Dip

Prep time: 5 minutes | Cook time: 5 minutes | Serves 4

- 1 small avocado
- 12 oz.cooked edamame beans
- 1/2 onion, chopped.
- 1/2 cup low-fat greek yogurt
- juice of a lemon

1. Mash the avocado and edamame beans with a fork until smooth.
2. Stir in the onions, Greek yogurt, and lemon juice.
3. Serve immediately.

PER SERVING

Calories: 120 kcal | Protein: 9g | Carbohydrates: 11g | Fat: 5g | Cholesterol: 0mg | Fiber: 4g

Cherry Tomato Bruschetta

Prep time: 15 minutes | Cook time: 15 minutes | Serves 4

- 8 ounces assorted cherry tomatoes, halved
- ⅓ cup fresh herbs, chopped (such as basil, parsley, tarragon, dill)
- 1 tablespoon extra-virgin olive oil
- ¼ teaspoon kosher salt
- ⅛ teaspoon freshly ground black pepper
- ¼ cup ricotta cheese
- 4 slices whole-wheat bread, toasted

1. Combine the tomatoes, herbs, olive oil, salt, and black pepper in a medium bowl and mix gently.
2. Spread 1 tablespoon of ricotta cheese onto each slice of toast. Spoon one-quarter of the tomato mixture onto each bruschetta. If desired, garnish with more herbs.

PER SERVING

Calories: 100 | Total fat: 6g | Saturated fat: 1g | Cholesterol: 5mg | Sodium: 135mg | Potassium: 210mg | Total Carbohydrates: 10g | Fiber: 2g | Sugars: 2g | Protein: 4g | Magnesium: 22mg | Calcium: 60mg

Turkey Cocktail Meatballs

Prep time: 20 minutes | Cook time: 1 hour 10 minutes | Serves 15

- 1-pound ground turkey breast
- 1/4 cup egg substitute
- 3/4 cup saltine crackers, crushed
- 4 ounces' part-skim shredded mozzarella
- 1/4 cup chopped onion
- 1/2 teaspoon ground ginger
- 6 tablespoons dijon mustard, divided
- 1 1/4 cups unsweetened pineapple juice
- 1/4 cup chopped green bell pepper
- tablespoons honey
- 1 tablespoon cornstarch

1. Preheat oven to 350°F (180°C, or gas mark 4).
2. Combine egg substitute, turkey, cracker crumbs, onion, ginger, mozzarella, and 3 tablespoons of mustard—form 30 balls out of the mixture, 1 inch (2.5 cm) each.
3. Spray a 9 x 13-inch (23 x 33-cm) baking dish with nonstick vegetable oil spray—place meatballs in the container. Bake, uncovered, for 20 to 25 minutes, or until cooked through.
4. Combine pineapple juice, green pepper, honey, cornstarch, onion powder, and remaining mustard in a saucepan.
5. Bring to a boil, stirring constantly. Cook and stir until thickened.

PER SERVING

Calories: 100 kcal | Protein: 10g | Carbohydrates: 9g | Fat: 2g | Cholesterol: 24mg | Fiber: 0g

Roasted Red Pepper Hummus

Prep time: 15 minutes | Cook time: 15 minutes | Makes about 2 cups

- 1 (15-ounce) can low-sodium chickpeas, drained and rinsed
- 3 ounces jarred roasted red bell peppers, drained
- 3 tablespoons tahini
- 3 tablespoons lemon juice
- 1 garlic clove, peeled
- ¾ teaspoon kosher salt
- ¼ teaspoon freshly ground black pepper
- 3 tablespoons extra-virgin olive oil
- ¼ teaspoon cayenne pepper (optional)
- Fresh herbs, chopped, for garnish (optional)

1. In a food processor, add the chickpeas, red bell peppers, tahini, lemon juice, garlic, salt, and black pepper.
2. Pulse 5 to 7 times. Add the olive oil and process until smooth. Add the cayenne pepper and garnish with chopped herbs, if desired.

PER SERVING

Calories: 130 | Total fat: 8g | Saturated fat: 1g | Cholesterol: 0mg | Sodium: 150mg | Potassium: 125mg | Total Carbohydrates: 11g | Fiber: 2g | Sugars: 1g | Protein: 4g | Magnesium: 20mg | Calcium: 48mg

Mango Popsicles

Prep time: 10 minutes | Cook time: 5 minutes | Serves 6

- 2 mangoes, peeled & diced
- 2 tbsp maple syrup
- 1 lime juice
- 14 oz can coconut milk

1. Add mangoes, maple syrup, lime juice, and coconut milk into the blender and blend until smooth.
2. Pour mango mixture into the popsicle molds and place in the refrigerator until set.
3. Serve chilled and enjoy.

PER SERVING

Calories: 221 | Fat:14.6 g | Carbohydrates: 24.6 g | Sugar: 21.2 g | Protein: 2.3 g | Cholesterol: 0 mg

Apple Crunch

Prep time: 10 minutes | Cook time: 45 minutes | Serves 6

For Apples:

- 4 apples, peeled, cored, and chopped
- 1/2 cup sugar
- 1 teaspoon cinnamon
- 1 tablespoon unsalted margarine

For Topping:

- 1/2 cup flour
- 1/2 cup sugar
- 1 teaspoon baking powder
- 1/4 cup egg substitute
- 1/2 cup sugar
- 1 tablespoon unsalted margarine

1. Preheat an oven to 350°F (180°C, or gas mark 4) to make the apples.
2. Mix apples, sugar, and cinnamon; pour into a greased 8 x 8-inch (20 x 20-cm) baking dish.
3. Dot with margarine.
4. To make the topping: Mix topping and pour over apples.
5. Bake for 30 to 35 minutes.

PER SERVING

Calories: 317 kcal | Protein: 3g | Carbohydrates: 70g | Fat: 4g | Cholesterol: 0mg | Fiber: 2 g

Healthy Summer Yogurt

Prep time: 10 minutes | Cook time: 5 minutes | Serves 6

- 2 cups frozen berries
- 1 tsp vanilla
- ½ cup Greek yogurt
- 2 tbsp maple syrup
- 2 frozen bananas

1. Add all ingredients into the blender and blend until smooth.
2. Pour blended mixture into the air-tight container, cover, and place in the freezer for 3 hours.
3. Serve chilled and enjoy.

PER SERVING

Calories: 99 | Fat:1.2 g | Carbohydrates: 18.9 g | Sugar: 14.8 g | Protein: 3 g | Cholesterol: 4 mg

Easy Pizza

Prep time: 10 minutes | Cook time: 40 minutes | Serves 16

- 1/2 cup unsalted margarine
- 3/4 cup brown sugar
- 1 egg yolk
- 1 teaspoon vanilla
- 1 1/2 cups flour
- 1 1/4 cups chocolate chips
- 1 1/2 cups miniature marshmallows
- 1/2 cup dry-roasted peanuts, chopped

1. Preheat oven to 350°F (180°C, or gas mark 4).
2. Beat the margarine in a large mixing bowl with an electric mixer on medium-high speed for 30 seconds.
3. Add brown sugar and beat until combined.
4. Beat in egg yolk and vanilla until combined.
5. Beat in as much of the flour as you can with the mixer.
6. Stir in any remaining flour with a wooden spoon.
7. Spread dough in a lightly greased 12-inch (30-cm) pizza pan.
8. Bake for 25 minutes, or until golden.
9. Sprinkle hot crust with the chocolate chips.
10. Let stand for 1 to 2 minutes to soften.
11. Spread chocolate over crust.
12. Sprinkle with marshmallows and nuts.
13. Bake for 3 minutes more or until marshmallows are puffed and brown.
14. Cool in pan on a wire rack.

PER SERVING

Calories: 247 kcal | Protein: 4g | Carbohydrates: 32g | Fat: 12g | Cholesterol: 16mg | Fiber: 1 g

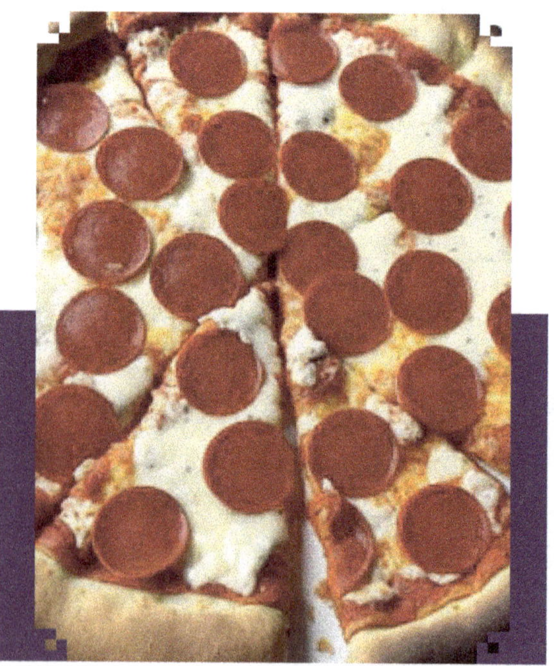

Chapter 6

Salads

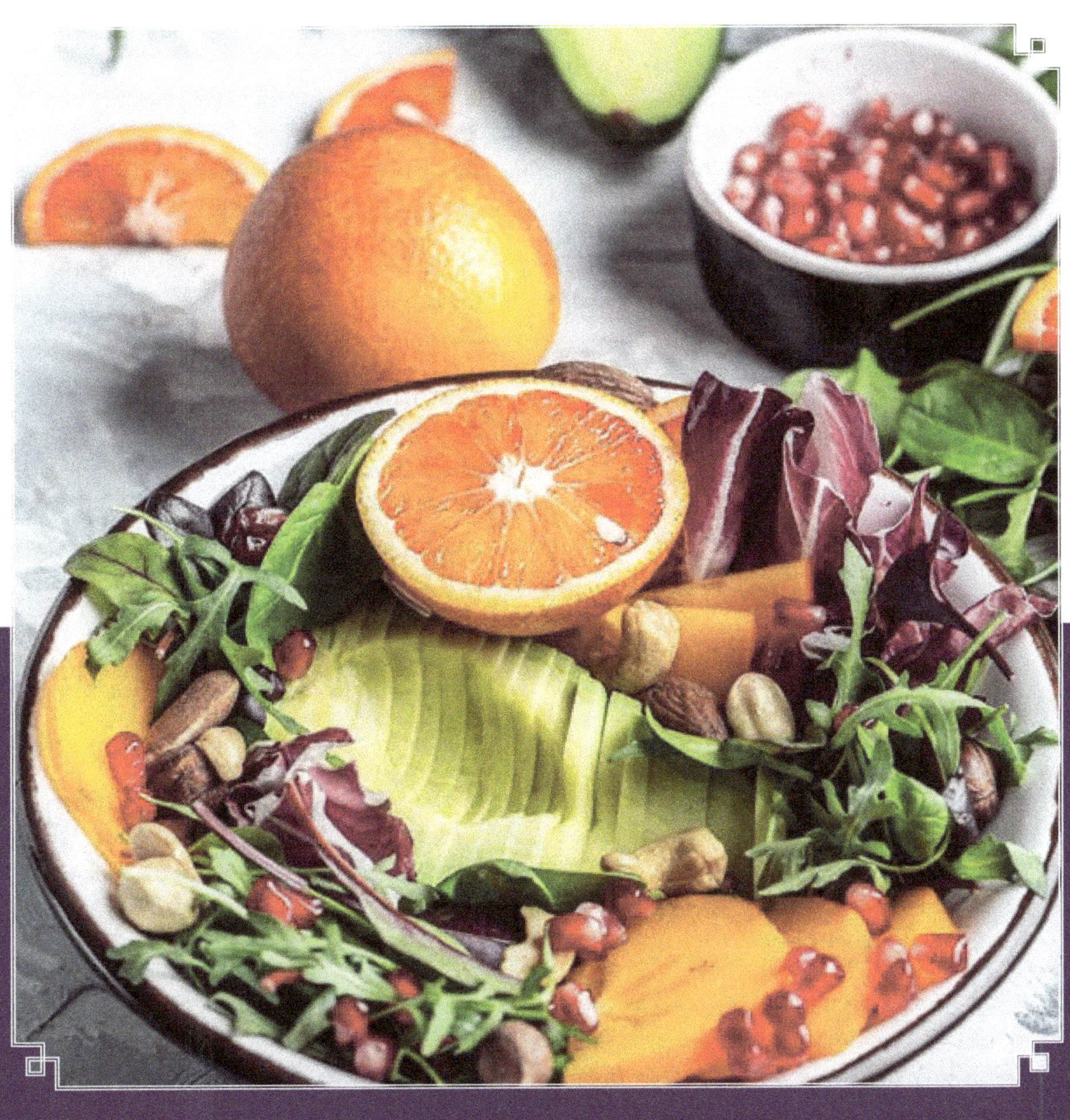

Tomato & Feta Salad

Prep time: 15 minutes | Cook time: 0 minutes | Serves 2

- 1 large fresh tomato, sliced
- ½ tablespoon olive oil
- 1 scallions, chopped
- 1½ tablespoon Feta cheese, crumbled
- 3 cups fresh baby greens
- ½ red onion, sliced
- 1 tablespoon unsalted almonds, chopped
- 1 tablespoon fresh lemon-juice

1. Take a bowl and add all the given ingredients except for almonds and cheese and toss to coat well.
2. Cover and refrigerate to let it sit and marinate for about six to eight hours.
3. Remove from the refrigerator and stir in the almonds.
4. Serve with the topping of Feta cheese.

PER SERVING

Calories: 150 | Fat: 6.8g | Sat Fat: 1.8g | Carbohydrates: 18.3g | Fiber: 6.8g | Sugar: 4.3g | Protein: 7.4g

Chicken & Strawberry Salad

Prep time: 10 minutes | Cook time: 16 minutes | Serves 4

- 4 tablespoons olive oil
- 1 tablespoon Erythritol
- 2 cups fresh strawberries
- 1 pound boneless, skinless chicken breasts
- 4 tablespoons lemon juice
- ½ garlic clove, minced
- 4 cups fresh spinach, torn
- Pinch of salt
- Fresh ground black pepper to taste

1. For marinade: Take a large bowl and add oil, lemon juice, Erythritol, garlic, salt and black pepper and beat them well until well combined.
2. In a large resalable plastic bag place chicken and ¾ cup marinade.
3. Seal the bag and shake it to coat well. Refrigerate overnight.
4. Cover the bowl of remaining marinade and refrigerate before serving.
5. Preheat the grill to medium heat.
6. Grease the grill grate finely.
7. Remove the chicken from bag and discard the marinade.
8. Place the chicken onto grill grate and grill it covered for about five to eight minutes per side.
9. Remove chicken from grill and cut into small pieces.
10. Take a large bowl, add the chicken pieces, strawberries and spinach and mix everything together.
11. Place the reserved marinade and toss to coat well.
12. Serve immediately and enjoy!

PER SERVING

Calories: 370 | Fat: 22.9g | Sat Fat: 4.5g | Carbohydrates: 10.8g | Fiber: 2.2g | Sugar: 7.7g | Protein: 34.3g

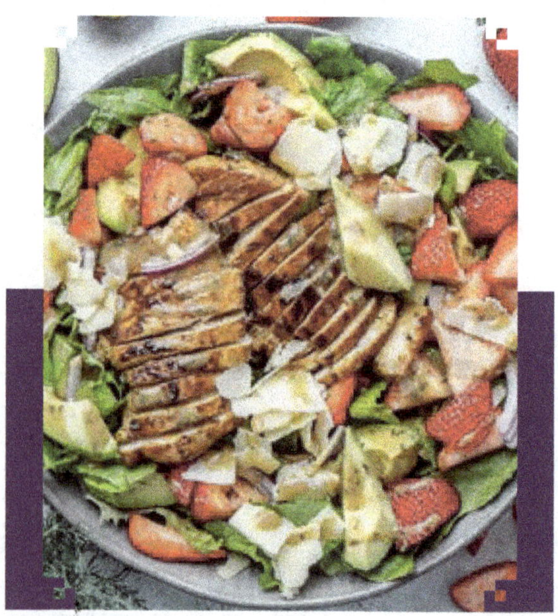

Salmon Couscous Salad

Prep time: 10 minutes | Cook time: 10 minutes | Serves 1

- ¼ cup sliced cremini mushrooms
- ¼ cup diced eggplant
- 3 cups baby spinach
- 2 tbsp. white-wine vinaigrette, divided
- ¼ cup cooked Israeli couscous, preferably whole-wheat
- 4 oz. cooked salmon
- ¼ cup sliced dried apricots
- 2 tbsp. crumbled goat's cheese (½ oz.)

1. Coat a small skillet with cooking spray and heat over medium-high heat. Add the mushrooms and eggplant. Cook, stirring, until lightly browned and the juices have been released (3 to 5 minutes). Remove from the heat and set aside.
2. Toss the spinach with 1 tbsp. plus 1 tsp. of vinaigrette and place on a 9-inch plate.

PER SERVING

Calories: 464 | Protein: 34.8g | Carbohydrates 34.7g | Dietary fiber 5.9g | Sugars 18.9g | Fat: 22.1g | Sodium: 352.1mg

Waldorf Chicken Salad

Prep time: 20 minutes | Cook time: 12 minutes | Serves 4

- ¼ cup plain nonfat greek yogurt
- 2 tablespoons mayonnaise
- 2 tablespoons dijon mustard
- 1 tablespoon honey
- ¼ teaspoon kosher or sea salt
- ¼ teaspoon ground black pepper
- 3 cups chopped cooked chicken breast
- 1 apple, diced
- 2 celery stalks, diced
- 1 cup green or red seedless grapes, halved
- ¼ cup chopped walnuts

1. In a bowl, whisk together the yogurt, mayonnaise, Dijon mustard, honey, salt, and black pepper.
2. Fold in the cooked chicken, apple, celery, grapes, and walnuts.
3. Store in airtight containers in the refrigerator for up to 3 days.

PER SERVING:

Total Calories: 353 | Total Fat: 14g | Saturated Fat: 2g | Cholesterol: 92mg | Sodium: 475mg | Potassium: 283mg | Total Carbohydrate: 20g | Fiber: 2g | Sugars: 17g | Protein: 36g

Zucchini and Brussels Sprouts Salad

Prep time: 10 minutes | Cook time: 3 hours | Serves 4

- 1-pound zucchinis, roughly cubed
- ½ pound Brussels sprouts, trimmed and halved
- ¼ cup veggie stock, low-sodium
- 1 teaspoon cumin, ground
- 1 teaspoon chili powder
- 2 teaspoon avocado oil

1. In a slow cooker, mix the sprouts with zucchini and other ingredients.
2. Cover, and simmer for 3 hours on low.
3. Divide between plates and serve as a side dish.

PER SERVING

Calories: 51 | Fat: 0.9 g | Sodium: 42 mg | Carbs: 9.8 g | Fiber: 3.8 g | Sugar: 3.3 g | Protein: 3.5 g

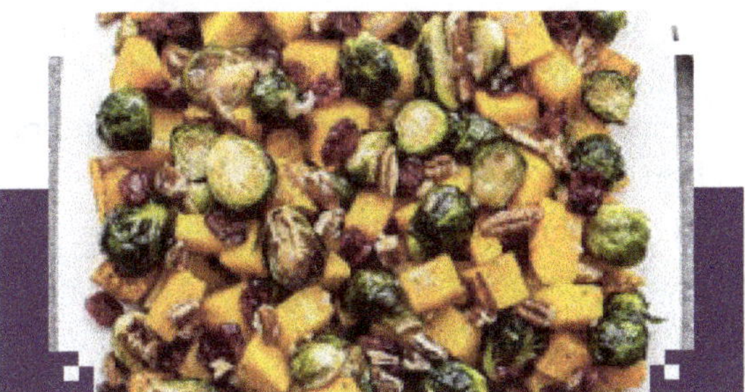

Mexican Bean Salad

Prep time: 10 minutes | Cook time: 10 minutes | Serves 8

- 2 cups cooked kidney beans
- 2 cups cooked garbanzo beans
- 1 cup tomatoes, chopped
- 3/4 cup cucumber, peeled & chopped
- 4 cups lettuce, shredded
- 1/2 cup avocado, mashed
- 2 tablespoons onion, diced
- 1/2 cup plain fat-free yogurt
- 1/4 teaspoon minced garlic
- 1/2 teaspoon cumin

1. Toss together the kidney beans, garbanzo beans, tomatoes, cucumber, and onion in a large bowl.
2. Mix the avocado, yogurt, garlic, and cumin in a small bowl.
3. Stir the avocado mixture into the bean mixture and chill.
4. Serve on top of shredded lettuce.

PER SERVING

Calories: 172 kcal | Protein: 9g | Carbohydrates: 29g | Fat: 3g | Cholesterol: 0mg | Fiber: 7g

Mandarin Almond Salad

Prep time: 20 minutes | Cook time: 40 minutes | Serves 8

- 6 thinly sliced green onions,
- 2 (11 ounces) cans of mandarin oranges, drained
- ½ cup of sliced almonds
- 2 tablespoons of white sugar
- ½ cup of olive oil
- 1 rinsed, dried, chopped head romaine lettuce -
- ¼ cup of red wine vinegar
- 1 tablespoon of white sugar
- ground black pepper; to taste.
- ⅛ teaspoon of red pepper flakes; crushed.

1. Combine the oranges, romaine lettuce, and green onions in a large mixing dish.
2. In a skillet over medium heat, melt 2 tablespoons of sugar with the almonds.
3. Cook and whisk until the sugar melts and coats the almonds.
4. Continually stir until the nuts are light brown.
5. Place on a platter and set aside to cool for almost 10 minutes.

PER SERVING

Calories: 235 kcal | Protein: 2g | Carbohydrates: 20.2g | Fat: 16.7g | Cholesterol: 0mg | Fiber: 1.8g

Fig and Goat's Cheese Salad

Prep time: 10 minutes | Cook time: 10 minutes | Serves 1

- 2 cups mixed salad greens
- 4 dried figs, stemmed and sliced
- 1 oz. fresh goat's cheese, crumbled
- 1½ tbsp. slivered almonds, preferably toasted
- 2 tsp. extra-virgin olive oil
- 2 tsp. balsamic vinegar
- ½ tsp. honey
- Pinch of salt
- Freshly ground pepper to taste

1. Combine the greens, figs, goat's cheese, and almonds in a medium bowl.
2. Stir together the oil, vinegar, honey, salt, and pepper.

PER SERVING

Calories: 340 | Protein: 10.4g | Carbohydrates 31.8g | Dietary fiber 7g | Sugars 21.8g | Fat: 21g | Sodium: 309.5mg

Chapter 7

Soups and Stews

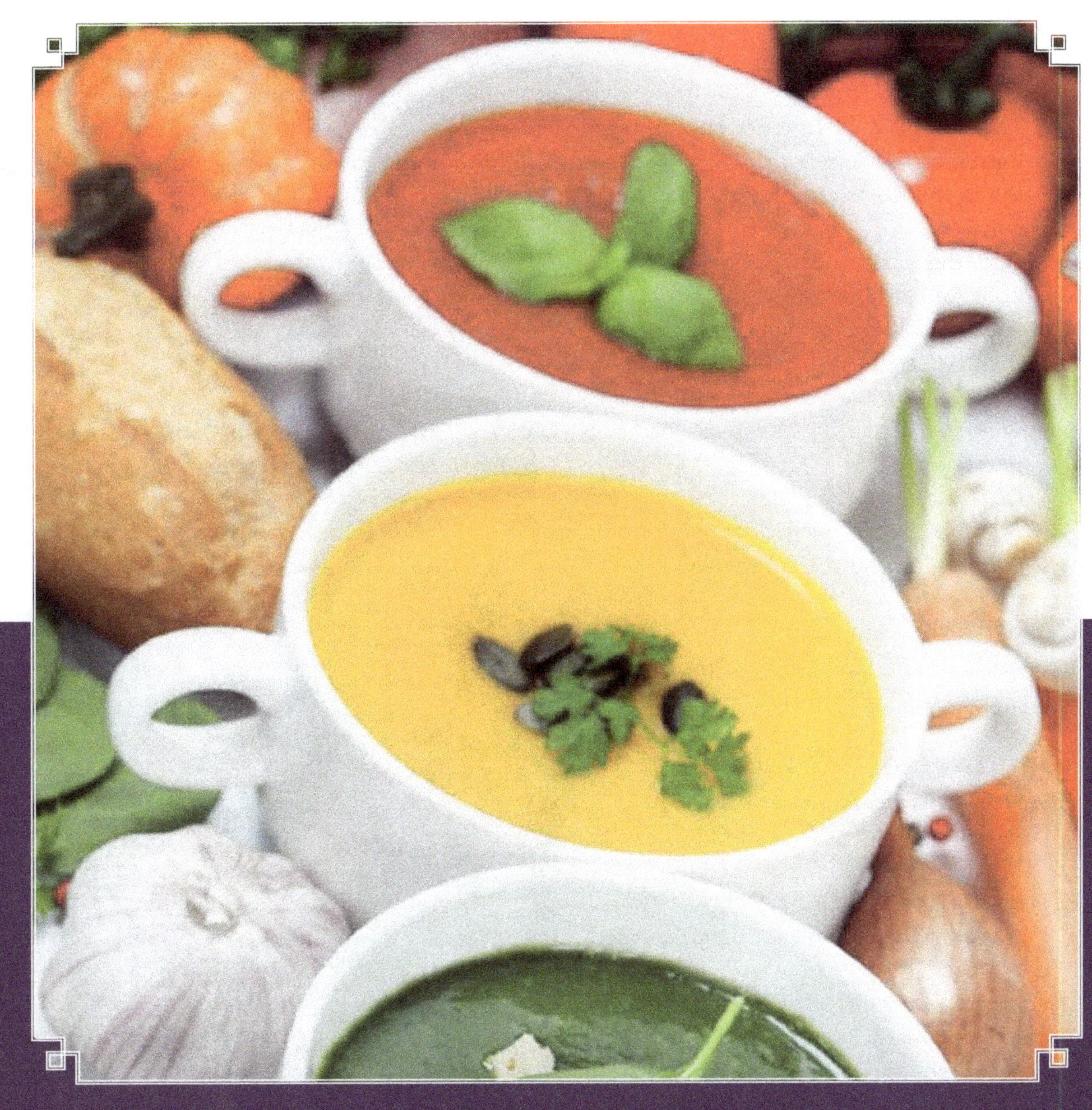

Linguini Chicken Soup

Prep time: 10 minutes | Cook time: 20 minutes | Serves 6

- 1 teaspoon olive oil
- 1 cup onion, chopped
- 3 garlic cloves, minced
- 1 cup celery, chopped
- 1 cup carrots, sliced and peeled
- 4 cups chicken broth
- 4 ounces dried linguini, broken
- 1 cup cooked chicken breast, cut into the desired size
- 2 tablespoons fresh parsley

1. Add the olive oil to a saucepan, then heat it on medium flame.
2. Stir in the garlic and onion. Sauté until soft.
3. Add the carrots and celery. Stir and cook for 3 minutes.
4. Pour in the broth and cook until it boils, then reduce it to a simmer.
5. Cook for 5 minutes, then add the linguini.
6. Bring to a boil and then reduce the heat to a simmer.
7. Cook for 10 more minutes.
8. Add the chicken and parsley.
9. Cook for a minute, then serve warm.

PER SERVING

Calories: 381 | Fat: 15g |Sodium 42mg | Carbs: 9.7g | Fiber: 0.4g | Sugar: 1g | Protein: 25.2g

Tomato Peach Soup

Prep time: 10 minutes | Cook time: 12 minutes | Serves 4

- ½ tablespoon olive oil
- 1 large ripe peach, halved, pitted, peeled and diced
- 1 cup carrots, shredded
- 2 garlic cloves, minced
- 1 can no-salt diced tomatoes in juice
- ½ teaspoon chili pepper, freshly ground
- 1 cup chicken broth, low-sodium
- 1 cup water
- 1 cup yogurt

1. Heat the olive oil in a large pot over medium heat.
2. Add the shredded carrots and cook, often stirring, about 5 minutes, or until carrots are tender. Sprinkle with garlic, and cook for 1 minute.
3. Remove the carrot mixture to a food processor.
4. Add the tomatoes and their juice, broth, chili pepper and water, and purée until smooth.
5. Return the purée to the pot, reduce heat to medium-low, cook the soup mixture for 5 minutes, or cook until cooked through.
6. Smear with the yogurt.
7. Enjoy.

PER SERVING

Calories: 155 | Fat: 9g | Sodium: 116mg | Carbs: 17g | Fiber: 5g | Sugar: 4g | Protein: 5g

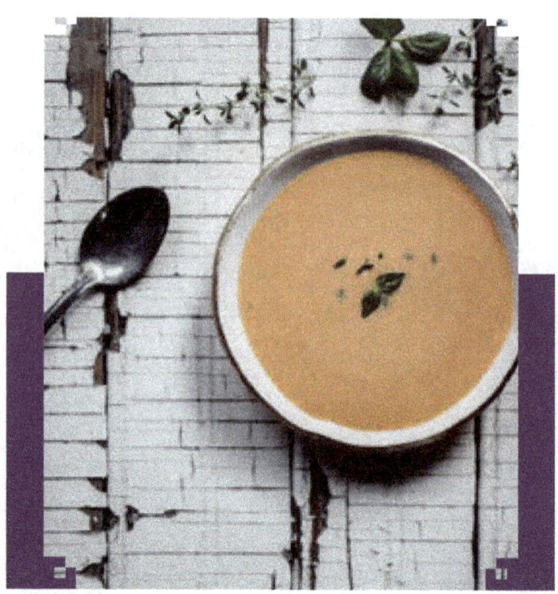

Slow-Cooked Mediterranean Chicken and Chickpea Soup

Prep time: 4 hours 20 minutes | Cook time: 20 minutes | Serves 6

- 1½ cups dried chickpeas, soaked overnight
- 4 cups water
- 1 large yellow onion, finely chopped
- 1 (15 oz.) can no-salt-added diced tomatoes, preferably fire-roasted
- 2 tbsp. tomato paste
- 4 cloves garlic, finely chopped
- 1 bay leaf
- 4 tsp. ground cumin
- 4 tsp. paprika
- ¼ tsp. cayenne pepper
- ¼ tsp. ground pepper
- 2 lbs. bone-in chicken thighs, skin removed, trimmed
- 1 (14 oz.) can artichoke hearts, drained and quartered
- ¼ cup halved pitted oil-cured olives
- ½ tsp. salt
- ¼ cup chopped fresh parsley or cilantro

1. Drain the chickpeas and place them in a 6-quart (or larger) slow cooker. Add 4 cups water, onion, tomatoes and their juice, tomato paste, garlic, bay leaf, cumin, paprika, cayenne, and ground pepper. Stir to combine.
2. Add the chicken.
3. Cover and cook on low for 8 hours or on high for 4 hours.
4. Transfer the chicken to a clean cutting board and let it cool slightly. Discard the bay leaf.
5. Add the artichokes, olives, and salt to the slow cooker and stir to combine.
6. Shred the chicken, discarding the bones. Stir the chicken back into the soup.

PER SERVING

Calories: 447 | Protein: 33.6g | Carbohydrates 43g | Dietary fiber 11.6g | Sugars 8.5g | Fat: 15.3g | Sodium: 761.8mg

Asparagus Soup

Prep time: 10 minutes | Cook time: 40 minutes | Serves 2

- ½ tablespoon olive oil
- ¾ pound asparagus, trimmed and chopped
- 1½ scallions, chopped
- 2 cups low-sodium vegetable broth
- 1 tablespoon fresh lemon juice
- ½ Serrano pepper, seeded and chopped finely

1. Take a large frying-pan and heat the oil over medium heat and fry the scallion for about four to five minutes.
2. Stir in the asparagus and broth and bring it to a boil.
3. Reduce the heat to low and let it cook for about 25-30 minutes while covered.
4. Remove the pan from the heat and set aside to let it cool.
5. Now, transfer the soup into a food processor in two batches and pulse until we have a smooth mixture.
6. Transfer the soup into the same pan over medium-heat and cook for about four to five minutes.
7. Stir in the lemon juice, salt and black pepper and remove from the heat.
8. Serve hot.

PER SERVING

Calories: 85 | Fat: 3.8g | Sat Fat: 0.6g | Carbohydrates: 8.7g | Fiber: 4g | Sugar: 3.7g | Protein: 6g

Chicken Barley Soup

Prep time: 10 minutes 1 hour 25 minutes | Cook time: 1 hour 35 minutes | Serves 5

- 1/2 cup of medium pearl barley
- 1 (2 to 3 pounds) broiler/fryer chicken, cut up
- 1 cup chopped celery.
- 1/2 teaspoon of pepper
- 8 cups of water
- 1-1/2 cups of chopped carrots
- 1 teaspoon of chicken bouillon granules
- 1/2 cup of chopped onion
- 1 teaspoon of salt, optional
- 1/2 teaspoon of rubbed sage.
- 1/2 teaspoon of poultry seasoning
- 1 bay leaf

1. Cook chicken in water in a large stockpot until tender.
2. Remove the fat from the soup once it has cooled.
3. Remove the chicken and set it aside until it is cold enough to handle.
4. Remove the flesh from the bones, toss out the bones, and chop the meat into cubes.
5. Return the meat, along with the other , to the pan.
6. Bring the water to a boil.
7. Reduce the heat to low, cover, and cook for 1 hour, or until the veggies and barley are soft.
8. Bay leaf should be discarded.

PER SERVING

Calories: 259 kcal | Protein: 31g | Carbohydrates:22g | Fat:5g | Cholesterol: 44mg | Fiber: 6 g

Brunswick Stew

Prep time: 10 minutes 1 hour 20 minutes | Cook time: 1 hour 30 minutes | Serves 8

- 15 ounces of low sodium tomato, canned.
- 4 cups of water
- 1 medium chopped onion,
- 2 skinless, boneless chicken breasts
- 15 ounces of butter beans
- 2 teaspoons of vegetable oil
- 15 ounces of corn

1. Boil four cups of water. Cook for 30 minutes, until chicken breasts are cooked through.
2. Allow the chicken to cool in the broth.
3. Cut it into bite-size pieces when the chicken has cooled enough to handle.
4. Using paper towels, spoon, or ice cubes, skim the fat from the chicken stock.
5. Soup can be made using broth.
6. Take 8 cups and measure them.
7. The remainder of the stock can be used for anything else.
8. Remove the brown layers from the onion by cutting the ends off.
9. Cut into small bits using a chef's knife.
10. In a large saucepan, heat the oil until it is very hot.
11. Add and cook until the onions are soft.
12. Add and cook for 30 minutes, or until chicken, butterbeans, tomatoes with their juices, and corn are cooked.

PER SERVING

Calories: 257 kcal | Protein: 25g | Carbohydrates: 34g | Fat: 4g | Cholesterol: 36mg | Fiber: 5g

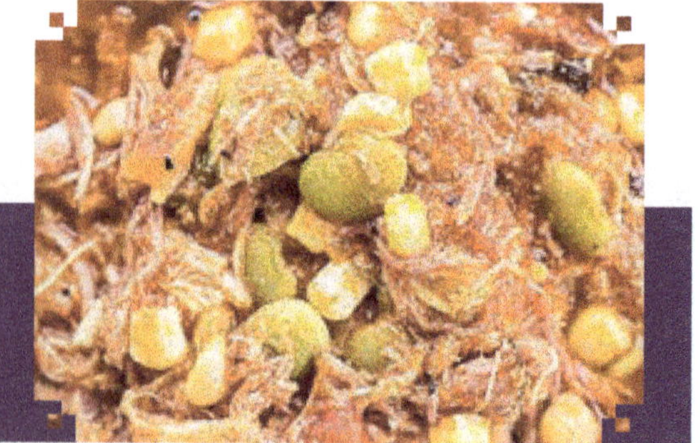

Chapter 8

Poultry

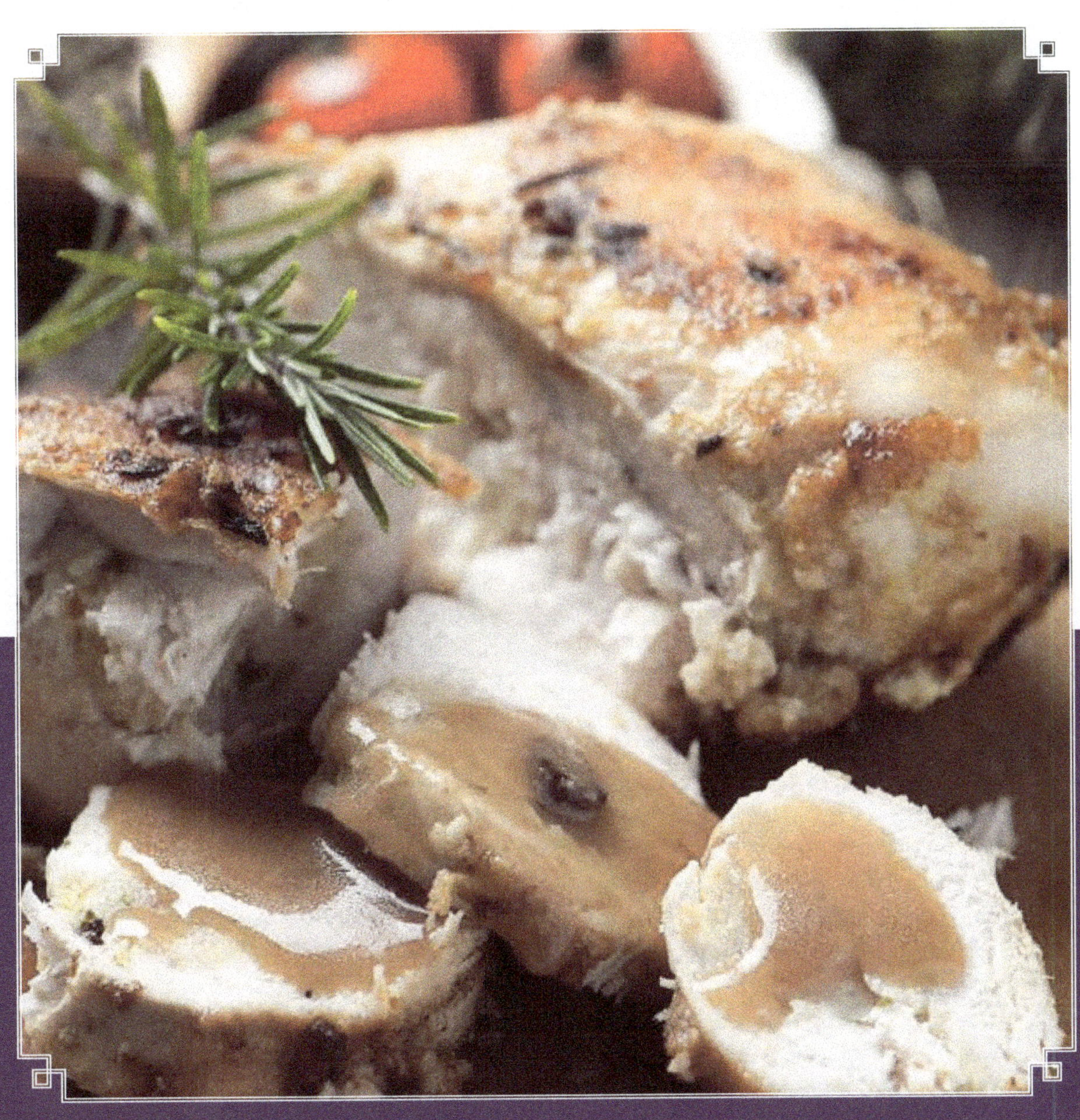

Chicken-Apricot Casserole

Prep time: 10 minutes | Cook time: 1 hour 5 minutes | Serves 4

- 2 chopped garlic cloves,
- 1 sliced onion,
- 2 teaspoons of ground cumin
- 8 chicken thighs,
- 1 1/4 cup of chicken broth; reduced-sodium.
- 2 tsp of ground coriander
- 5 pitted and quartered apricots,
- 2 tbsp of canola oil
- 3 carrots, halved crosswise, 6 to 8 thick fingers,
- chopped fennel leaves.
- salt and pepper to taste.

1. Fennel should be split lengthwise and then cut crosswise into slices on a cutting board.
2. In a large pan, heat the oil and cook the chicken thighs, flipping periodically, until golden brown on both sides, for about 5 to 10 minutes.
3. Remove it from the pan.
4. Sauté the garlic and onion in the pan for approximately 5 minutes, or until tender and golden.
5. Add all of the spices and cook for 1 minute before adding the stock.
6. Return the chicken and the fennel and carrots to the pan.
7. Bring the water to a boil.
8. Stir thoroughly, then cover and cook for 30 minutes, or until the chicken is cooked.
9. Take off the cover.
10. If there is too much liquid, decrease it somewhat by boiling.
11. Stir the apricots into the casserole gently to blend.
12. Cook for another 5 minutes over low heat.
13. Season with salt and pepper to taste.
14. Serve with a sprinkling of fennel leaves.

PER SERVING

calories: 280 kcal | Protein: 26g | Carbohydrates: 18g | Fat: 13g | Cholesterol: 49.5mg | Fiber: 0.7g

Chicken and Spaghetti Bake

Prep time: 10 minutes | Cook time: 45 minutes | Serves 6

- 8 ounces spaghetti
- 1/2 cup egg substitute
- 1 cup fat-free cottage cheese
- 1-pound boneless chicken breast, sliced
- 1/2 cup onion, chopped
- 1/2 cup green bell pepper, chopped
- 2 cups canned no-salt-added tomatoes
- 6 ounces no-salt-added tomato paste
- 1 teaspoon sugar
- 1 teaspoon dried oregano
- 1/2 teaspoon garlic powder
- 1/2 cup mozzarella, shredded

1. Preheat oven to 350°F (180°C, or gas mark 4).
2. Cook spaghetti to package directions.
3. Drain.
4. Mix in egg substitute.
5. Form into a "crust" in a greased 10-inch (25-cm) pie pan.
6. Top with cottage cheese.
7. In a large skillet, cook chicken, onion, and green bell pepper until meat is done and vegetables are tender.
8. Add remaining except for mozzarella and heat through.
9. Spread over spaghetti and cottage cheese. Bake for 20 minutes.
10. Sprinkle with mozzarella about 5 minutes before the end of baking.

PER SERVING

Calories: 218 kcal | Protein: 27g | Carbohydrates: 22g | Fat: 2g | Cholesterol: 46mg | Fiber: 4g

Harissa Yogurt Chicken Thighs

Prep time: 5 minutes, plus 15 minutes to marinate | Cook time: 25 minutes | Serves 4

- ½ cup plain Greek yogurt
- 2 tablespoons harissa
- 1 tablespoon lemon juice
- ½ teaspoon kosher salt
- ¼ teaspoon freshly ground black pepper
- 1½ pounds boneless, skinless chicken thighs

1. In a bowl, combine the yogurt, harissa, lemon juice, salt, and black pepper. Add the chicken and mix together. Marinate for at least 15 minutes, and up to 4 hours in the refrigerator.
2. Preheat the oven to 425°F. Line a baking sheet with parchment paper or foil. Remove the chicken thighs from the marinade and arrange in a single layer on the baking sheet. Roast for 20 minutes, turning the chicken over halfway.
3. Change the oven temperature to broil. Broil the chicken until golden brown in spots, 2 to 3 minutes.

PER SERVING

Calories: 190 | Total fat: 10g | Saturated fat: 2g | Cholesterol: 107mg | Sodium: 230mg | Potassium: 300mg | Total Carbohydrates: 1g | Fiber: 0g | Sugars: 1g | Protein: 24g | Magnesium: 28mg | Calcium: 24mg

Basil Pesto Chicken

Prep time: 10 minutes | Cook time: 15 minutes | Serves 4

- 8 oz uncooked rotini pasta
- 1 lb. asparagus, woody ends removed, cut into bite-size pieces
- 1 tbsp coconut oil
- 2 medium Roma tomatoes, chopped
- ½ cup basil pesto
- 12 oz boneless, cut into bite-size cubes, skinless chicken breasts
- ¼ cup Parmesan cheese, grated

1. Follow the package directions for cooking the rotini pasta or al dente. Scoop out ½ cup of the cooking water, and keep to one side. Add the asparagus pieces to the pasta when it reaches the remaining 4 minutes. Allow boiling.
2. Heat the coconut oil over medium-high heat in a large, heavy-bottom pan. Fry the cubed chicken breasts for 5 to 10 minutes or until cooked through. Stir in the chopped tomatoes, and remove the pan from the heat.
3. Drain the pasta and asparagus in a colander, and return them to the stockpot.
4. Toss the pasta and asparagus with the basil pesto and ¼ cup of the reserved cooking water. Add the cooked chicken mixture and more cooking water if needed.
5. Top with the grated Parmesan cheese, and serve hot.

PER SERVING

Calories: 485 | Total Fat: 17g | Saturated Fat: 4g | Cholesterol: 68mg | Sodium: 201mg | Total Carbs: 50g | Fiber: 5g | Protein: 33g

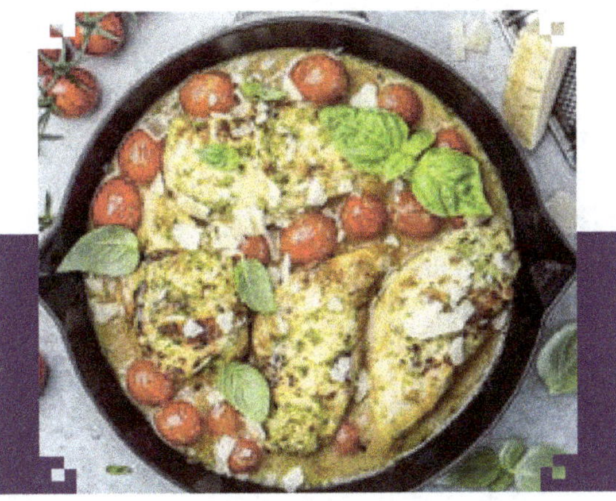

Olive Turkey Patties

Prep time: 10 minutes | Cook time: 30 minutes | Serves 4

- Aluminum foil
- 1 lb. lean ground turkey
- ½ cup rolled oats
- ¼ cup sliced black olives, chopped
- ¼ cup white onion, finely chopped
- ¼ cup parsley, finely chopped
- 1 tbsp garlic, minced
- 6 whole-wheat hamburger buns
- 1 ripe avocado, peeled, pitted, and sliced
- 6 iceberg lettuce leaves
- 6 beefsteak tomato slices

1. Preheat the broiler and set a baking sheet about 3 inches from the heat source. Line a baking sheet with aluminum foil.
2. In a large mixing bowl, add the ground turkey, rolled oats, chopped black olives, chopped onion, chopped parsley, and minced garlic. Mix well until combined. Shape into 6 equal patties.
3. Place the turkey patties on the baking sheet, and broil for 3 to 4 minutes on each side, or until the juices run clear.
4. Meanwhile, place the whole-wheat buns, sliced avocado, iceberg lettuce, and tomato slices on a serving platter. Allow diners to assemble their burgers.

PER SERVING

Calories: 366 | Total Fat: 15g | Saturated Fat: 3g | Cholesterol: 52mg | Sodium: 353mg | Total Carbs: 35g | Fiber: 6g | Protein: 24g

Balsamic Berry Chicken

Prep time: 10 minutes | Cook time: 30 minutes | Serves 2

- Aluminum foil
- ½ cup blueberries
- 2 tbsp pine nuts
- ¼ cup basil, finely chopped
- 2 tbsp balsamic vinegar
- ¼ tsp ground black pepper
- 2 (4 oz) chicken breasts, butterflied

1. Heat the oven to 375F, gas mark 5. Line a medium-sized baking dish with aluminum foil.
2. Add together the blueberries, pine nuts, chopped basil, balsamic vinegar, and ground black pepper in a medium-sized mixing bowl. Mix until well combined.
3. Place the chicken pieces in the pan, and pour the blueberry mixture on top.
4. Bake for 20 to 30 minutes, or until the juices are caramelized, and the inside of the chicken is fully cooked.
5. Serve warm with a side dish of your choice.

PER SERVING

Calories: 212 | Total Fat: 7g | Saturated Fat: 1g | Cholesterol: 80mg | Sodium: 58mg | Total Carbs: 11g; Net Carbs: 7g | Fiber: 2g | Protein: 27g

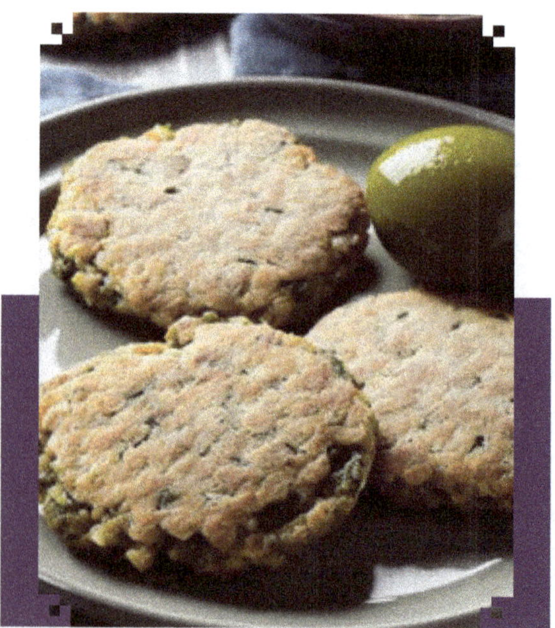

Moroccan Chicken

Prep time:15 minutes | Cook time: 20 minutes | Serves 4

- 3 (4-ounce) boneless, skinless chicken thighs, cubed
- 1 teaspoon smoked paprika
- ½ teaspoon ground cinnamon
- ½ teaspoon ground cumin
- ⅛ teaspoon ground ginger
- 1 cup low-sodium chicken broth
- 2 tablespoons fresh lemon juice
- 1 tablespoon cornstarch
- 1 teaspoon olive oil
- 1 onion, chopped
- 3 cloves garlic, minced
- 2 cups sugar snap peas
- 1 cup shredded carrots

1. Put the cubed chicken in a medium bowl. Sprinkle with the paprika, cinnamon, cumin, and ginger, and work the spices into the meat. Set aside.
2. In a small bowl, combine the chicken broth, lemon juice, and cornstarch and mix well. Set aside.
3. Heat the olive oil in a large nonstick skillet over medium-high heat. Add the chicken thighs, and sauté for 5 minutes or until the chicken starts to brown. Remove the chicken from the pan and set aside.
4. Add the onion and garlic to the skillet, and sauté for 3 minutes.
5. Add the sugar snap peas and carrots to the skillet and sauté for 2 minutes.
6. Return the chicken to the skillet and stir. Add the chicken broth mixture, bring to a simmer, and turn down the heat to low. Simmer 3 to 4 minutes or until the sauce thickens, the vegetables are tender, and the chicken is cooked to 165°F on a meat thermometer. Serve hot.

PER SERVING

Calories: 165 | Fat: 5g | Saturated Fat: 1g | Monounsaturated Fat: 3g | Carbs: 11g | Sodium: 112mg | Dietary Fiber: 3g | Protein: 18g | Cholesterol: 70mg | Vitamin A: 267% DV | Vitamin C: 67% DV | Sugar: 4g

Mini Turkey Meatloaves

Prep time:10 minutes | Cook time: 20 minutes | Serves 4

- ⅓ cup old-fashioned rolled oats
- 2 scallions, finely chopped
- 1 egg
- 3 tablespoons no-salt-added tomato paste, divided
- 2 teaspoons olive oil
- pinch salt
- ⅛ teaspoon black pepper
- ½ teaspoon dried ground leaves
- 16 ounces 99% lean ground white turkey
- 2 tablespoons low-sodium mustard
- 1 tablespoon water

1. Preheat the oven to 450°F. Line a baking sheet with aluminum foil.
2. In a large bowl, combine the oats, scallions, egg, 2 tablespoons of the tomato paste, olive oil, salt, pepper, and marjoram, and mix well.
3. Add the ground turkey, and mix gently with your hands until well combined.
4. Divide the mixture into fourths and shape into mini loaves. Place on the prepared baking sheet.

PER SERVING

Calories: 205 | Fat: 5g | Saturated Fat: 1g | Monounsaturated Fat: 0g | Carbs: 8g | Sodium: 252mg | Dietary Fiber: 1g | Protein: 30g | Cholesterol: 111mg | Vitamin A: 4% DV | Vitamin C: 4% DV | Sugar: 1g

Chapter 9

Meat

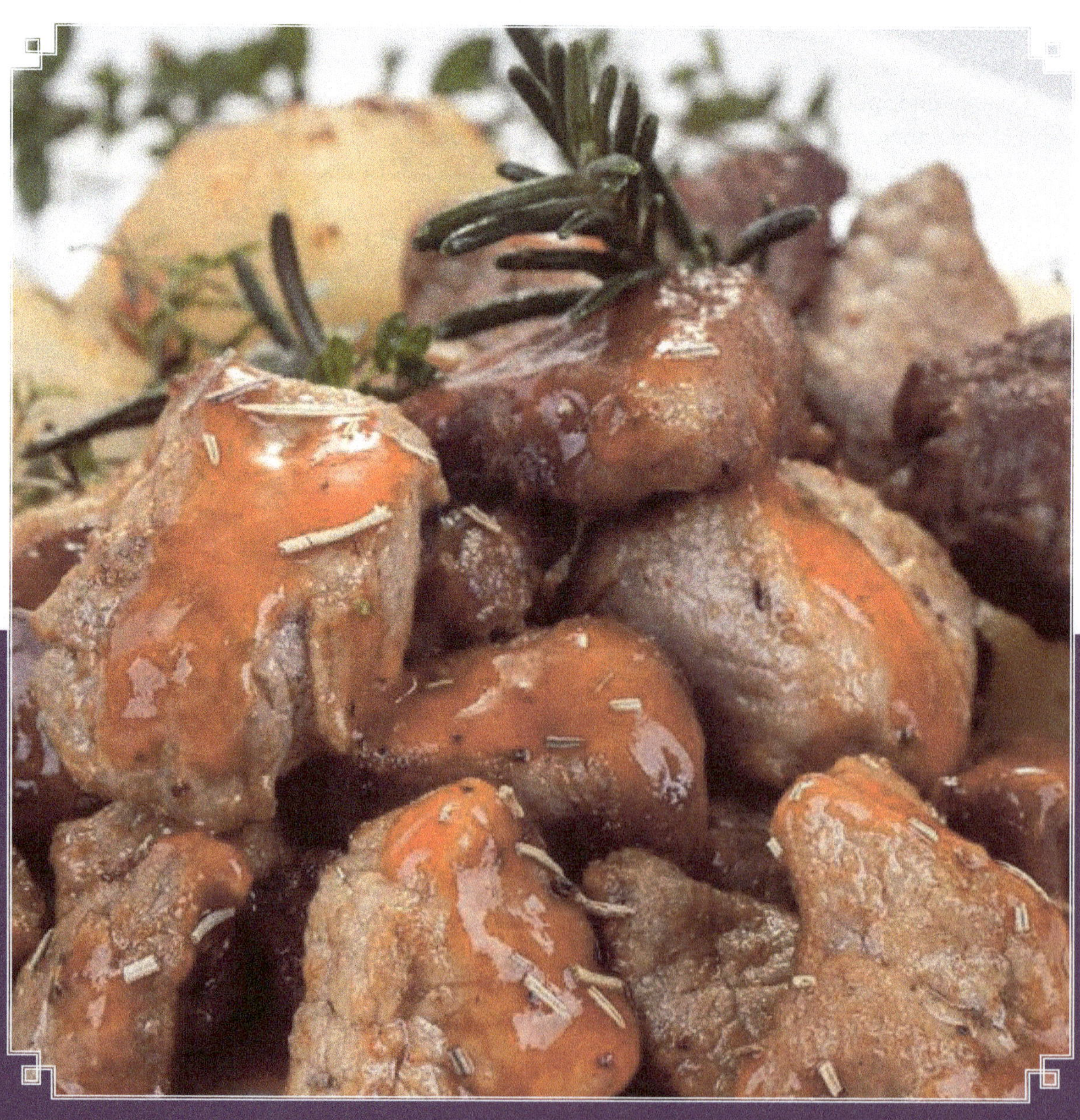

Bbq Pulled Pork with Greek Yogurt Slaw

Prep time: 10 minutes 1 hour | Cook time: 1 hour 10 minutes | Serves 4

- 3 cups of green cabbage; shredded
- 1/2 cup of non-fat plain greek yogurt
- 3 cups of red cabbage; shredded
- 1 (12oz.) can of diet root beer
- 2 tsp of lemon juice
- 1 tbsp. of apple cider vinegar
- 1/4 tsp of celery salt
- 1 tsp of dijon mustard
- 1 can of light cooking spray
- 1 1/2 lbs. pork tenderloin; halved
- 1 pinch stevia
- 4 sachets of buttermilk cheddar herb biscuit
- 1/2 cup of bbq sauce; sugar-free

1. Cooking spray is used to coat the interior of the Instant Pot.
2. On a high sauté ' setting, brown the pork chunks on all sides, approximately 3 minutes on each side.
3. Close the pressure valve after adding the diet root beer. Set the timer for 60 minutes on high. Allow for natural pressure release before opening.
4. Prepare the slaw in the meanwhile. Combine cabbage, yogurt, apple cider vinegar, lemon juice, Dijon mustard, salt, and stevia in a medium-sized mixing bowl.
5. Remove the pork from the Instant Pot and shred it in a bowl.
6. Toss in the barbecue sauce and mix well. Bake Herb Biscuits according to package instructions, if desired. Serve the slaw and shredded pork on top of biscuits or without baked biscuits.

PER SERVING

Calories: 108 kcal | Protein: 5.8g | Carbohydrates: 14g | Fat: 2.5g | Cholesterol: 39.9mg | Fiber: 3.5g

Lemon Garlic Flank Steak Wraps

Prep time:15 minutes | Cook time: 15 minutes | Serves 4

- ½ pound flank steak
- ⅛ teaspoon garlic powder
- pinch salt
- ⅛ teaspoon lemon pepper
- 3 tablespoons fresh lemon juice
- 1 tablespoon orange juice
- 1 red bell pepper, seeded and sliced
- 1 cucumber, sliced
- 3 stalks celery, sliced
- 2 cups fresh baby spinach
- 4 (8-inch) whole-wheat flour tortillas

1. In a shallow bowl, sprinkle the flank steak with the garlic powder, salt, and lemon pepper. Drizzle all over with the lemon juice and orange juice and let stand for 10 minutes while you prepare the rest of the ingredients.
2. Heat a grill pan or nonstick skillet over medium-high heat. Add the steak, and cook 5 to 6 minutes per side, turning once, until cooked to at least 145°F on a meat thermometer.
3. Remove the steak from the grill and let rest for 2 minutes. Cut the steak across the grain into thin slices.
4. Divide the steak, vegetables, and spinach, among the 4 tortillas. Roll up, tucking in the ends, cut in half, and serve.

PER SERVING

Calories: 292 | Fat: 9g | Saturated Fat: 4g | Monounsaturated Fat: 0g | Carbs: 31g | Sodium: 513mg | Dietary Fiber: 2g | Protein: 21g | Cholesterol: 40mg | Vitamin A: 40% DV | Vitamin C: 87% DV | Sugar: 4g

Bavarian Beef

Prep time: 10 minutes | Cook time: 2 hours 20 minutes | Serves 5

- 1 tbsp of vegetable oil
- 1/8 tsp of black pepper
- 1/2 small head of red cabbage, 4 wedges
- 1 1/4 lb. of lean beef/; stew meat, remove fat: 1-inch pieces.
- 1/4 cup of crushed gingersnaps,
- 1 large thinly sliced onion,
- 1 1/2 cup of water
- 3/4 tsp of caraway seeds
- 1/2 tsp of salt
- 1/4 cup of white vinegar
- 1 bay leaf
- 1 tbsp of sugar

1. In a large skillet, brown the meat in the oil.
2. Remove the meat and cook the onion until golden in the remaining oil.
3. Return the meat to the pan.
4. Water, pepper, salt, caraway seeds, and bay leaf are added to the pot.
5. Bring it to a boil.
6. Reduce the heat to low, cover, and cook for 1 1/4 hours.
7. Stir in the sugar and vinegar.
8. On top of the meat, arrange the cabbage.

PER SERVING

Calories: 218 kcal | Protein: 24g | Carbohydrates: 14g | Fat: 7g | Cholesterol: 60mg | Fiber: 1 g

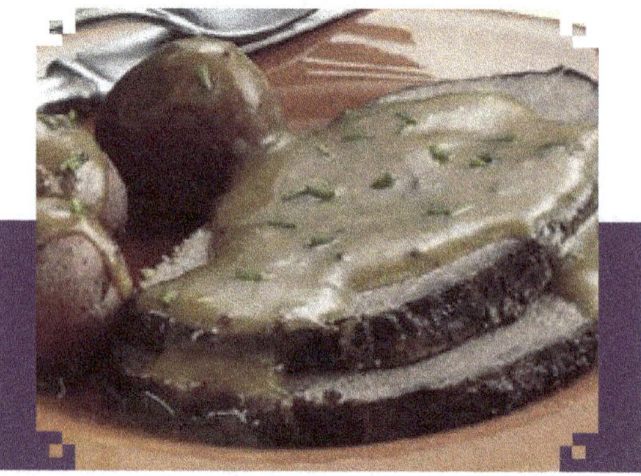

Spicy Sichuan Orange Beef Vegetable Stir-Fry

Prep time: 10 minutes | Cook time: 12 minutes | Serves 2

- ¾ cup orange juice
- 1 tablespoon reduced-sodium soy sauce
- 1 tablespoon unseasoned rice vinegar or dry sherry
- 1 teaspoon sesame oil
- 2 teaspoons cornstarch
- ¼ teaspoon chinese five-spice powder
- 1 teaspoon red pepper flakes
- 2 teaspoons extra-virgin olive oil
- 8 ounces boneless beef sirloin steak, cut into thin strips
- 3 cloves garlic, minced
- 2 teaspoons grated fresh ginger
- 3 cups frozen stir-fry vegetable blend

1. In a small bowl, combine the orange juice, soy sauce, rice vinegar, sesame oil, cornstarch, five-spice, and pepper flakes until smooth. Set aside.
2. In a large skillet or wok, heat 1 teaspoon of the olive oil over high heat. Add the beef and stir-fry until no longer pink, 3 to 4 minutes. Remove with a slotted spoon to a plate; cover to keep warm.
3. Add the remaining 1 teaspoon olive oil to the pan. Add the garlic and ginger and stir-fry for 1 minute. Add the vegetables and continue cooking for 2 to 3 minutes, until thawed. Stir the sauce and pour into the pan, bring to a boil, and cook for 2 to 3 minutes to thicken. Return the beef to the pan, stir to combine, and cook for an additional 1 to 2 minutes to heat through.

PER SERVING

Calories: 321 | Total fat: 12 g | Saturated fat: 3 g | Cholesterol: 65 mg | Sodium: 376 mg | Potassium: 454 mg | Total carbohydrates: 22 g | Fiber: 4 g | Sugars: 13 g | Protein: 28 g

Shredded Beef Tacos

Prep time: 4 hours 30 minutes | Cook time: 7 hours | Serves 4

- 2 tablespoons of vinegar
- ¼ cup of vegetable oil
- 1 ½ teaspoon of ground cumin
- 2 tablespoons of lime juice
- 3 minced cloves of garlic,
- 1 ½ teaspoon of chili powder
- 1 ½ pound of beef chuck roast; trim it, 1-inch-thick slices
- salt to taste
- 1 cup of beef stock

1. Combine the vinegar, vegetable oil, lime juice, chili powder, cumin, and garlic; pour it into a resalable plastic bag.
2. Add the sliced beef to the bag, cover it with the marinade, press out any air, and close it.
3. Marinate for 4 hours or overnight in the refrigerator.
4. Preheat the oven to 350 degrees Fahrenheit (175 degrees C).
5. Place the meat with the lime juice marinade in a large baking dish.
6. Cover the baking dish with aluminum foil after adding the beef stock.
7. Bake it for 2 1/2 hours in a preheated oven until the meat is extremely tender.
8. Allow 20 minutes for the meat to come to room temperature.
9. Allow 10 minutes for the meat to rest before shredding with two forks.
10. Before serving, drain and discard approximately 80% of the liquid from the meat.

PER SERVING

Calories: 399 kcal | Protein: 21.2g | Carbohydrates: 3.1g | Fat: 33.3g | Cholesterol: 77.2mg | Fiber: 4g

Mediterranean Brisket

Prep time: 10 minutes | Cook time: 5 hours 40 minutes | Serves 8

- 3 teaspoons of dried crushed italian seasoning,
- 1 3-pound of fresh beef brisket
- 2 media trimmed, fennel bulbs, cored, and cut into wedges.
- ½ cup of beef broth; lower-sodium
- 1 (14.5 ounces) can have diced no-salt-added tomatoes with garlic, basil, and oregano, undrained
- ½ cup of pitted olives
- 1 cup of fresh italian parsley; (flat-leaf)
- ¼ teaspoon of salt
- 1 teaspoon of lemon peel; finely shredded
- ¼ teaspoon of ground black pepper
- 2 tablespoons of all-purpose flour
- ¼ cup of cold water

1. Trim any excess fat from the beef.
2. Season it with 1 teaspoon of Italian spice.
3. Place the meat in a slow cooker with a capacity of 3 1/2 to 4 quarts.
4. Fennel should be sprinkled on top.
5. Stir broth, salt, tomatoes, olives, pepper, lemon peel, and the remaining 2 teaspoons of Italian seasoning in a mixing bowl.
6. Pour everything into the cooker.
7. Cook on low heat for 10-11 hours or on high heat for 5 to 5 1/2 hours, covered.
8. Remove the meat from the cooker and set aside the juices.
9. Meat should be sliced.
10. Arrange the meat and veggies on a plate and keep them warm by covering them.

PER SERVING

Calories: 254 kcal | Protein: 34.8g | Carbohydrates: 10.2g | Fat: 8.4g | Cholesterol: 50.6mg | Fiber: 0.21 g

Steak with Red Onions, Peppers, and Mushrooms

Prep time: 5 minutes | Cook time: 12 minutes | Serves 2

- 8 ounces top round steak
- salt and freshly ground black pepper
- 4 teaspoons extra-virgin olive oil
- 2 cloves garlic, minced
- ½ medium red onion, sliced into rings
- 1 small red bell pepper, sliced into big chunks
- 1 small green bell pepper, sliced into big chunks
- 1 cup sliced baby bella mushrooms

1. Slice the beef into thin strips. Season with a dash each of salt and black pepper.
2. Heat a large skillet over high heat. When the skillet is hot, add 1 teaspoon of the olive oil and half of the beef. Cook 1 minute, then flip the steak strips and cook an additional 30 seconds. Set aside in a large dish.
3. Add another 1 teaspoon olive oil to the skillet and heat over high heat. Add the remaining steak, cook 1 minute, then flip and cook an additional 30 seconds. Set aside with the other cooked steak.
4. Add another 1 teaspoon olive oil to the skillet over high heat. Add the garlic, onion, and bell peppers and cook until the onion is golden and the peppers are soft, 3 to 4 minutes. Add the cooked vegetables to the dish with the steak.

PER SERVING

Calories: 293 | Total fat: 14 g | Saturated fat: 3 g | Cholesterol: 75 mg | Sodium: 76 mg | Potassium: 224 mg | Total carbohydrates: 12 g | Fiber: 2 g | Sugars: 5 g | Protein: 28 g

Italian Pot Roast

Prep time: 10 minutes | Cook time: 6 hours 35 minutes | Serves 8

- 6 whole peppercorns
- 1 cinnamon stick (3 inches)
- 3 whole allspice berries
- 4 whole cloves
- 1 (2 pounds) beef chuck roast; boneless
- 2 teaspoons of olive oil
- 2 medium sliced carrots,
- 2 sliced celery ribs,
- 4 minced garlic cloves,
- 1 large, chopped onion,
- 1 can of crushed tomatoes; (28 ounces)
- 1 cup of dry sherry or beef broth; reduced-sodium.
- hot egg noodles; cooked and minced parsley, optional
- 1/4 teaspoon of salt

1. Place the peppercorns, cloves, cinnamon stick, and allspice on a double layer of cheesecloth.
2. To enclose the spices, gather the corners of the fabric and bind them firmly with thread.
3. Heat the oil in a large skillet over medium-high heat.
4. Brown the roast on both sides and place it in a 4-quart slow cooker.
5. Add the carrots, celery, and spice bag to the pot.
6. In the same skillet, cook and sauté the onion until soft.
7. Cook for a further minute after adding the garlic.
8. Stir in the sherry to remove any browned pieces from the bottom of the pan.

PER SERVING

Calories: 251 kcal | Protein: 24g | Carbohydrates: 11g | Fat: 12g | Cholesterol: 74mg | Fiber: 2 g

Beef Tenderloin with Chickpeas and Artichoke Hearts

Prep time: 10 minutes | Cook time: 15 minutes | Serves 4

- 1 tablespoon extra-virgin olive oil
- 4 beef tenderloin filets (4 ounces each), trimmed of fat
- 4 cloves garlic, chopped
- pinch of red pepper flakes
- 4 cups baby spinach
- 1 (15-ounce) can chickpeas, rinsed and drained
- 1 (14-ounce) can water-packed artichoke hearts, drained and rinsed
- 1 cup chopped fresh tomatoes, with their juices
- 2 teaspoons dried marjoram
- ½ cup chopped fresh basil leaves
- salt and freshly ground black pepper (optional)

1. In a large sauté pan, heat the olive oil over medium-high heat until shimmering. Add the beef and cook until the filets are well browned on the bottom, about 2 minutes. Flip and cook until well browned on the second side, another 2 minutes. Transfer to a plate and cover to keep warm.
2. Reduce the heat under the skillet to medium. Add the garlic and sauté until golden brown, about 1 minute. Add the pepper flakes and spinach. Cook and stir for 1 minute to wilt the spinach. Add ½ cup water, then cover the pan and bring to a simmer. Uncover and cook until almost all of the water is evaporated, 3 to 4 minutes.
3. Add the chickpeas, artichoke hearts, tomatoes with their juices, and the marjoram. Cook for 2 minutes and stir to allow the sauce to coat the vegetables.
4. Return the beef to the pan along with any collected juices on the plate and toss in the fresh basil. Cover and cook until the beef is cooked to your desired doneness, 2 to 3 minutes.
5. Place a beef filet on each of 4 serving plates. Season the vegetables with salt and pepper, if desired, and portion onto the plates with the beef.

PER SERVING

Calories: 348 | Total fat: 11 g | Saturated fat: 3 g | Cholesterol: 60 mg | Sodium: 129 mg | Potassium: 1,054 mg | Total carbohydrates: 29 g | Fiber: 12 g | Sugars: 4 g | Protein: 34 g

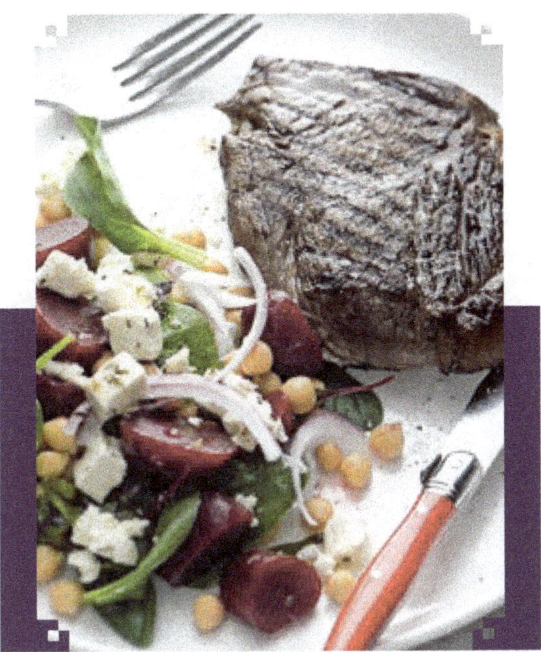

Chapter 10

Fish and Seafood

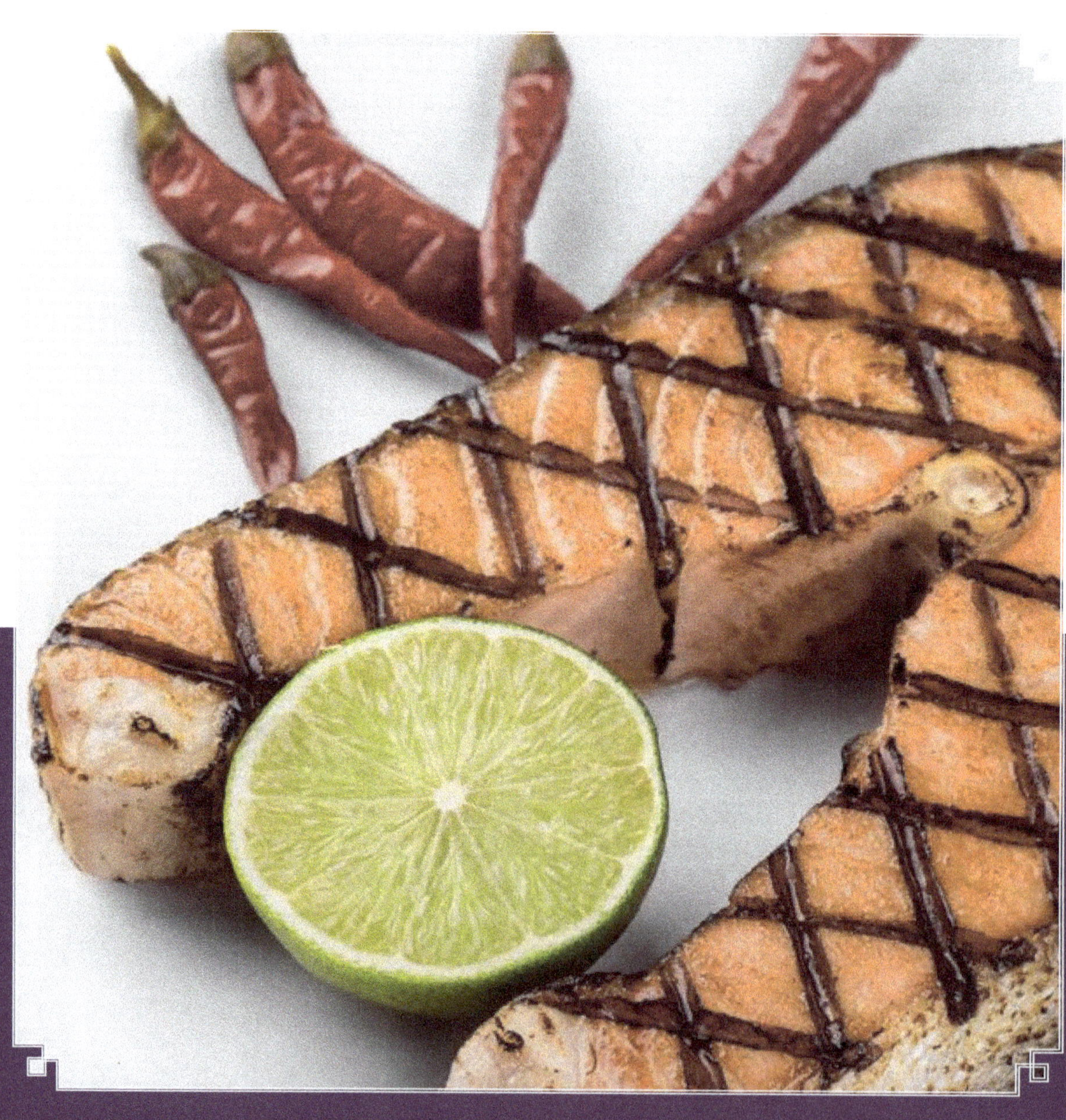

Fish Veracruz

Prep time: 20 minutes | Cook time: 50 minutes | Serves 8

- 1/2 tablespoon of canola oil
- 1/4 cup of lime juice
- 1 small peeled and sliced onion,
- 1/4 cup of seeded and sliced.
- 1 small seeded green bell pepper, strips
- 2 cups of pico de gallo or fresh salsa
- jalapeno pepper,
- 1/2 cup of tomato sauce; no salt added.
- 2 pounds of whitefish fillets, such as sole, tilapia, pollock cod, or halibut
- 1 tablespoon of capers
- 1/2 cup of sliced ripe olives
- 1 lime, 8 wedges
- 4 tablespoons of chopped fresh cilantro, / 4 teaspoons of dried cilantro.

1. In a baking pan of 9-by-13-inch, arrange the fish. Lime juice is sprinkled on top. Refrigerate it for 20 minutes after covering.
2. Preheat the oven to 425 degrees Fahrenheit. In a large non-stick skillet, heat the oil over medium-high heat. Add the bell pepper, onion, and jalapeño pepper.
3. Cook for 2 minutes, stirring periodically, or until veggies are cooked yet crisp.
4. Add salsa, olives, tomato sauce, and capers.
5. Bring it to a boil. Reduce heat to low and cook for 1 minute.
6. Pour sauce over the fish and bake for 20 minutes in a preheated oven or until the fish flakes easily with a fork.
7. with a slotted spatula, remove the fish and veggies from the pan. Serve with lime wedges and cilantro.

PER SERVING

Calories: 172 kcal | Protein: 23g | Carbohydrates: 11g | Fat: 4g | Cholesterol: 57mg | Fiber: 2.1g

Tuna Couscous

Prep time: 15 minutes | Cook time: 25 minutes | Serves 4

- 1 cup dry couscous
- 2 tablespoons olive oil
- 2 large carrots, thinly sliced
- 4 cups green beans, cut into 1-inch pieces
- 2 yellow zucchinis, sliced in half lengthwise and cut into half rounds
- sea salt for seasoning
- freshly ground black pepper for seasoning
- 2 (4-ounce) can chunk albacore tuna

1. Prepare the couscous according to package directions and set aside.
2. In a large skillet, heat the olive oil over medium-high heat.
3. Sauté the carrots until tender-crisp, about 5 minutes.
4. Add the green beans, zucchini, and sauté until the vegetables are tender about 5 minutes.
5. Season the vegetables with salt and pepper.
6. Spoon the couscous into 4 bowls and evenly divide the vegetables between them.
7. Serve topped with tuna.

PER SERVING

Calories: 357 kcal | Protein: 21g | Carbohydrates: 48g | Fat: 10g | Cholesterol: 25mg | Fiber: 8 g

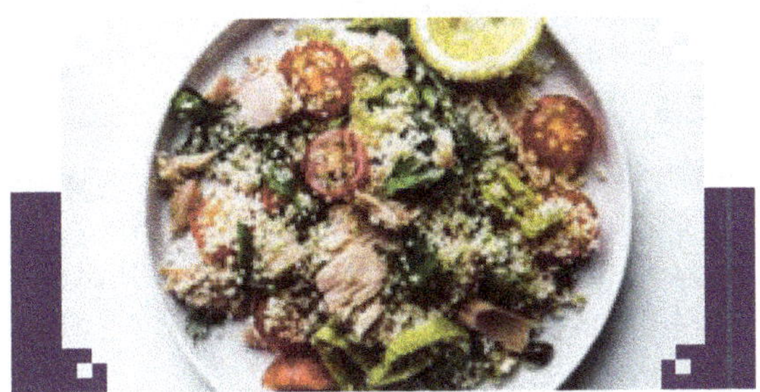

Cod Satay

Prep time: 15 minutes | Cook time: 15 minutes | Serves 4

- 2 teaspoons olive oil, divided
- 1 small onion, diced
- 2 cloves garlic, minced
- 1/3 cup low-fat coconut milk
- 1 tomato, chopped
- 2 tablespoons low-fat peanut butter
- 1 tablespoon packed brown sugar
- 1/3 cup low-sodium vegetable broth
- 2 teaspoons low-sodium soy sauce
- 1/8 teaspoon ground ginger
- Pinch red pepper flakes
- 4 (6-ounce) cod fillets
- 1/8 teaspoon white pepper

1. In a small saucepan, heat 1 teaspoon of the olive oil over medium heat.
2. Add the onion and garlic, and cook, stirring frequently for 3 minutes.
3. Add the coconut milk, tomato, peanut butter, brown sugar, broth, soy sauce, ginger, and red pepper flakes, and bring to a simmer, stirring with a whisk until the sauce combines. Simmer for 2 minutes, then remove the satay sauce from the heat and set aside.
4. Season the cod with the white pepper.
5. Heat a large nonstick skillet with the remaining 1 teaspoon olive oil, and add the cod fillets. Cook for 3 minutes, then turn and cook for 3 to 4 minutes more or until the fish flakes when tested with a fork.
6. Cover the fish with the satay sauce and serve immediately.

PER SERVING

Calories 255 | Fat: 10g | Saturated Fat: 5g | Monounsaturated Fat: 3g | Carbs:9g | Sodium: 222mg | Dietary Fiber: 1g | Protein: 33g | Cholesterol: 72mg | Vitamin A: 4% DV | Vitamin C: 9% DV | Sugar: 4g

Shrimp Pasta Primavera

Prep time: 20 minutes | Cook time: 40 minutes | Serves 6

- 12 ounces whole-grain spaghetti
- 1½ tablespoons unsalted butter
- 1 small head broccoli, chopped
- 1 red bell pepper, seeded and chopped
- 1 pound raw shrimp, deveined and shelled
- 1 cup frozen green peas
- 1 cup baby spinach leaves
- 5 garlic cloves, peeled and minced
- ¾ teaspoon kosher or sea salt
- ½ teaspoon ground black pepper
- ¼ teaspoon crushed red pepper flakes
- zest and juice of 1 lemon
- ½ cup unsalted vegetable, chicken, or fish stock
- ½ cup freshly grated parmesan cheese
- ¼ cup fresh flat-leaf italian parsley, chopped

1. Bring a large pot of water to a boil. Cook the spaghetti according to the package directions. Reserve ¼ cup of pasta water and drain the rest.
2. In a Dutch oven or large pot, heat the butter over medium heat. Add the broccoli and red bell pepper and sauté for 2 to 3 minutes, until slightly soft. Add the shrimp, green peas, and spinach and sauté for 2 to 3 minutes, until the shrimp is opaque. Stir in the garlic, salt, black pepper, and crushed red pepper flakes. Cook until fragrant.
3. Add the reserved pasta water, lemon zest and juice, and stock and bring to a simmer for 6 to 8 minutes, until thickened, stirring frequently.

PER SERVING:

Total Calories: 369 | Total Fat: 7g | Saturated Fat: 2g | Cholesterol: 125mg | Sodium: 546mg | Potassium: 469mg | Total Carbohydrate: 43g | Fiber: 9g | Sugars: 5g | Protein: 30g

Spinach & Feta Salmon Burgers

Prep time: 10 minutes | Cook time: 20 minutes | Serves 4

- 1 pound salmon fillets, skin removed
- 1 cup fresh spinach, chopped
- ½ cup panko bread crumbs
- ¼ cup crumbled feta cheese
- 1 large egg
- 1 tablespoon dijon mustard
- ½ teaspoon dried dill
- ¼ teaspoon kosher or sea salt
- ¼ teaspoon ground black pepper
- ½ cup plain nonfat greek yogurt
- ½ english cucumber, sliced
- 1 beefsteak tomato, sliced

1. Preheat the oven to 400°F. Line a baking sheet with parchment paper.
2. Place the salmon in the bowl of a food processor and pulse until ground. Transfer to a bowl and stir in the spinach, bread crumbs, feta cheese, egg, Dijon mustard, dill, salt, and black pepper until well combined. Use your hands to form 4 burger-size patties. Place them on the parchment paper and bake for 20 minutes, until the internal temperature reaches 145°F.
3. Serve the burgers with dollops of the Greek yogurt and slices of the cucumber and tomato.
4. For leftovers, place the burgers in microwaveable airtight containers for up to 3 to 4 days. Reheat in the microwave on high for 2 to 3 minutes, until heated through. Assemble the burgers before consuming.

PER SERVING:

Total Calories: 238 | Total Fat: 8g | Saturated Fat: 2g | Cholesterol: 109mg | Sodium: 453mg | Potassium: 106mg | Total Carbohydrate: 10g | Fiber: 1g | Sugars: 3g | Protein: 30g

Grilled Salmon with Chimichurri

Prep time: 15 minutes | Cook time: 10 minutes | Serves 4

- ½ cup fresh flat-leaf italian parsley leaves
- ¼ cup fresh cilantro leaves
- ½ jalapeño, seeded
- 4 cloves garlic, peeled
- ¼ cup red wine vinegar
- 2 tablespoons olive oil
- 1 teaspoon honey
- 1 teaspoon dried oregano leaves
- ½ teaspoon kosher or sea salt
- ¼ teaspoon ground black pepper
- 4 (4-ounce) salmon fillets, skin on
- 1 tablespoon olive oil
- 2 teaspoons chili powder

1. Preheat the grill to medium. Rub the salmon fillets with the olive oil and season with the chili powder, salt, and black pepper. Place the fillets on the grill, skin-side down, and cook about 10 minutes, until the fish flakes easily with a fork.
2. Serve the chimichurri over the grilled salmon fillets.

PER SERVING:

Total Calories: 341 | Total Fat: 25g | Saturated Fat: 5g | Cholesterol: 70mg | Sodium: 532mg | Potassium: 127mg | Total Carbohydrate: 4g | Fiber: 1g | Sugars: 2g | Protein: 26g

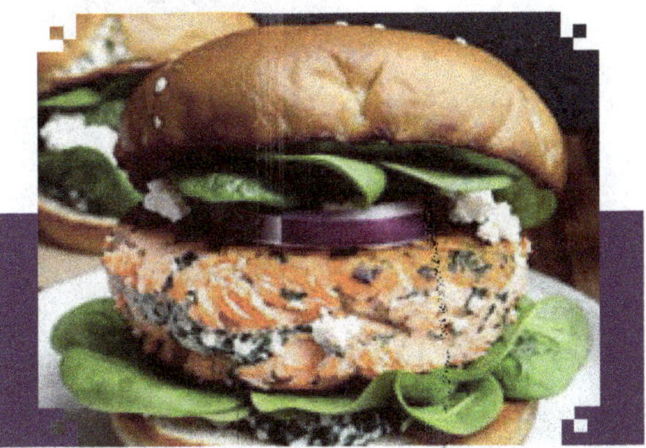

Chapter 11

Vegetarian and Vegan Recipes

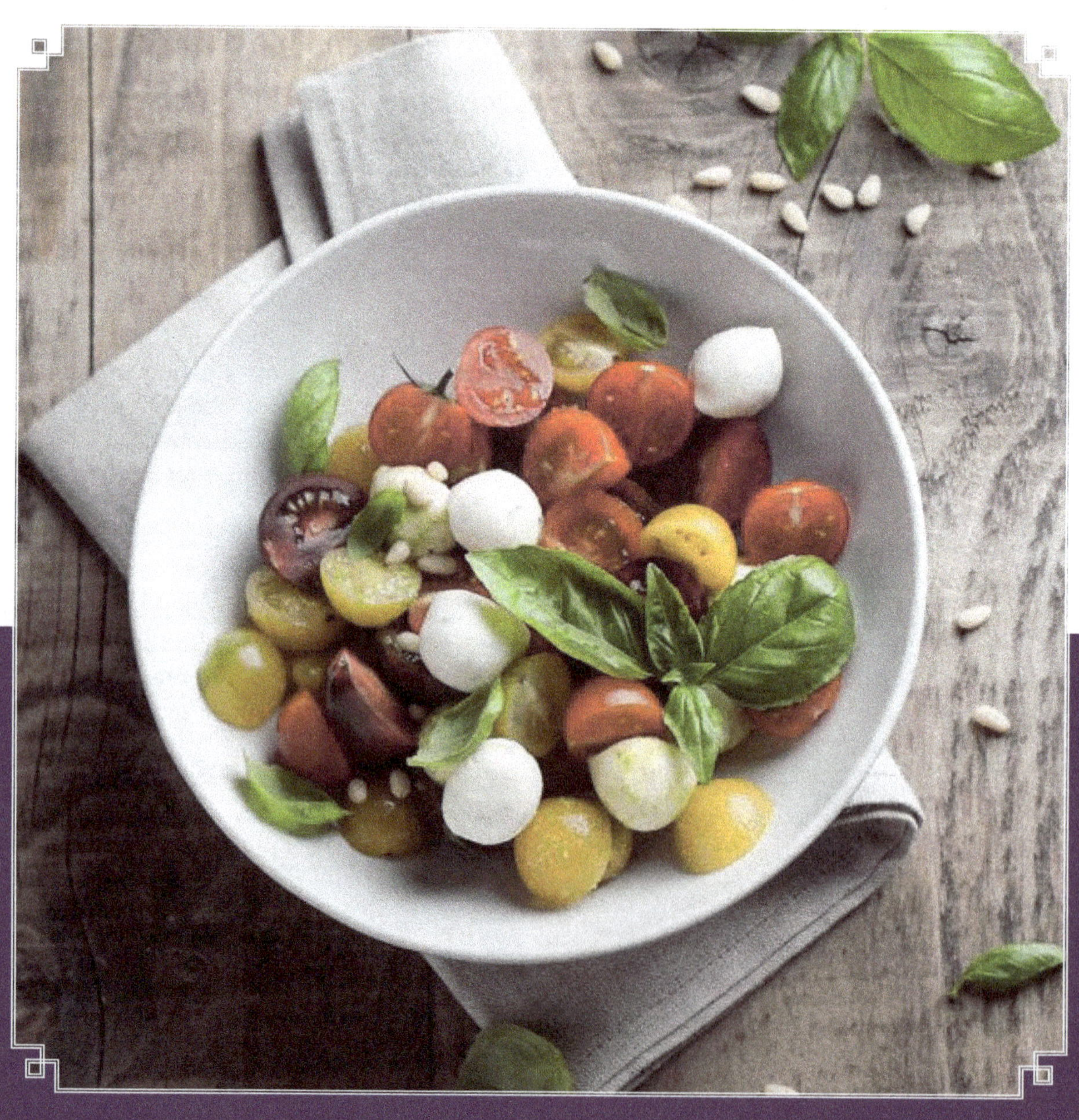

Roasted Red Pepper and Spinach Falafel

Prep time: 15 minutes | Cook time: 30 minutes | Serves 4

Falafel:

- 1 (15-ounce) can chickpeas, rinsed and drained
- ⅓ cup chopped red onion
- 4 cloves garlic, coarsely chopped
- ½ cup packed fresh parsley, destemmed
- ½ cup jarred roasted red peppers, drained
- 1 cup baby spinach
- 2 teaspoons ground cumin
- 2 teaspoons sweet paprika
- 1 teaspoon ground coriander
- 1 teaspoon freshly ground black pepper
- ⅛ teaspoon cayenne pepper
- ⅛ teaspoon salt
- 2 teaspoons extra-virgin olive oil
- 1 tablespoon fresh lemon juice
- about ¼ cup chickpea flour (or other flour)
- 2 tablespoons black or white sesame seeds (optional)

Tzatziki:

- ½ cup nonfat (0%) plain greek yogurt
- ⅓ cup peeled and grated cucumber
- 1 tablespoon minced fresh dill
- 1 teaspoon fresh lemon juice
- ¼ teaspoon minced garlic

1. Make the falafel: Preheat the oven to 375°F. Line a baking sheet with parchment paper.
2. In a food processor, combine the chickpeas, onion, garlic, parsley, roasted red peppers, spinach, cumin, paprika, coriander, black pepper, cayenne, salt, olive oil, and lemon juice. Pulse several times, then blend until fully incorporated but not entirely smooth, as you want a bit of texture.
3. Scoop out the falafel mixture into a large bowl and add the chickpea flour 1 tablespoon at a time until you have a workable dough that isn't too sticky but is still a bit wet.
4. Place the sesame seeds (if using) in a small bowl.
5. Using a large spoon, measure out portions of the mixture and form into golf ball-size balls (I usually get 12 balls but you can make as many or few as you like). If you are using the optional sesame seeds, roll the balls in the seeds. Place the falafel on the lined baking sheet and flatten them a bit with the palm of your hand.
6. Transfer to the oven and bake until browned, about 30 minutes, turning halfway through.
7. While the falafel are baking, make the tzatziki: In a small bowl, stir together the yogurt, cucumber, dill, lemon juice, and garlic. Refrigerate until ready to use.
8. Serve the falafel with the tzatziki sauce. These also make a great appetizer.

PER SERVING

Calories: 192 | Total fat: 4 g | Saturated fat: 1 g | Cholesterol: 1 mg | Sodium: 73 mg | Potassium: 411 mg | Total carbohydrates: 29 g | Fiber: 8 g | Sugars: 7 g | Protein: 11 g

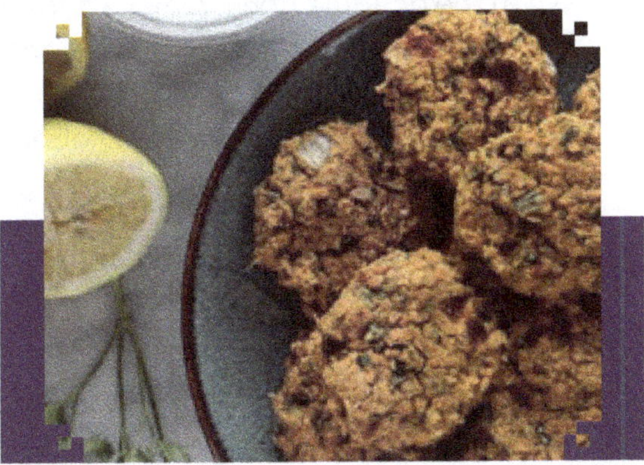

Roasted Vegetable Stuffed Pizza

Prep time: 20 minutes | Cook time: 1 hour 20 minutes | Serves 6

- 1 cup water
- 4 teaspoons olive oil
- 1 1/2 cups bread flour
- 1 1/2 cups whole wheat flour
- 1 1/2 teaspoons yeast
- 3 cups mushrooms, quartered
- 2 cups zucchini, sliced
- 1 cup onion, sliced
- 1 cup red bell pepper, sliced
- 1 cup green bell pepper, sliced
- 1 tablespoon olive oil

1. Preheat oven to 450°F (230°C, or gas mark 8).
2. Place the first 5 (through yeast) in a bread machine pan in the order specified by the manufacturer.
3. Process on the dough cycle.
4. Meanwhile, combine mushrooms, zucchini, onion, red and green bell peppers, and olive oil in a large baking pan.
5. Bake vegetable mixture for 20 minutes, or until tender and browned on the edges.
6. Stir in spaghetti sauce and set aside.
7. Reduce oven heat to 350°F (180°C, or gas mark 4).
8. Grease the bottom and sides of a 9-inch (23-cm) springform pan.
9. When the dough is done, remove it from the bread machine, punch down, and rest for 10 minutes.
10. Separate into two balls, with about three-quarters of the dough in the largest one.

PER SERVING

Calories: 393 kcal | Protein: 15g | Carbohydrates: 62g | Fat: 11g | Cholesterol: 9mg | Fiber: 8 g

Vegetarian Chili and Tofu

Prep time: 5 minutes | Cook time: 40 minutes | Serves 4

- 12 ounces of extra-firm tofu; small pieces
- 1 small chopped yellow onion (1/2 cup)
- 1 no salt added, can of kidney beans; rinsed and drained (14 ounces)
- 2 no added salt cans of diced tomatoes (14 ounces each)
- 1 tablespoon of olive oil
- 3 tablespoons of chili powder
- 1 no salt added can of black beans; rinsed and drained (14 ounces)
- 1 tablespoon of chopped fresh cilantro.
- 1 tablespoon of oregano

1. Heat olive oil in a soup pot over medium heat.
2. Add onions and cook for approximately 6 minutes, or until tender and transparent.
3. Add tomatoes, tofu, chili powder, beans, and oregano.
4. Cook it.
5. Reduce the heat to low and cook for at least 30 minutes.
6. Take the pan off the heat and toss in the cilantro.
7. Immediately ladle into separate bowls and serve.

PER SERVING

Calories: 314 kcal | Protein: 19g | Carbohydrates: 46g | Fat: 6g | Cholesterol: 0mg | Fiber: 4g

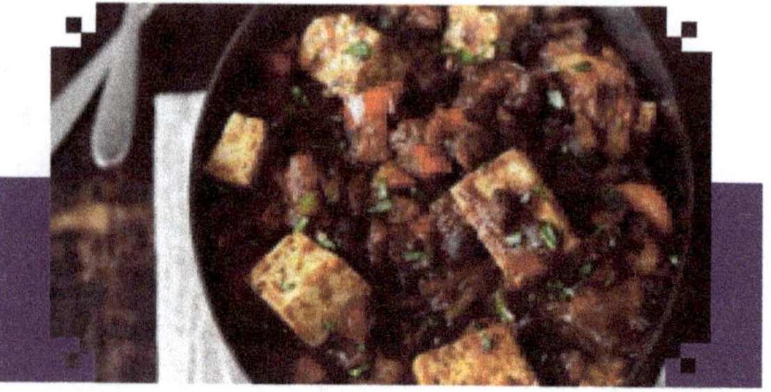

Bean and Tomato Curry

Prep time: 10 minutes | Cook time: 30 minutes | Serves 6

- 1 tablespoon canola oil
- 1 teaspoon mustard seed
- 1 teaspoon cumin seeds
- 1 cup onion, chopped
- 1 tablespoon fresh ginger, peeled and chopped
- 1/2 teaspoon chopped garlic
- 4 cups canned no-salt-added tomatoes
- 2 cups kidney beans, drained and rinsed
- 1 teaspoon curry powder

1. Heat oil in a large pot over medium heat and stir-fry the mustard and cumin seeds until they pop.
2. Add onion, ginger, and garlic, and stir-fry until lightly colored.
3. Add tomatoes with juice, beans, and curry powder.
4. Simmer for about 20 minutes or until thick and saucy.

PER SERVING

Calories: 140 kcal | Protein: 7 g | Carbohydrates: 23 g | Fat: 3 g | Cholesterol: 0 mg | Fiber: 6 g

Coconut Rice and White Beans

Prep time: 10 minutes | Cook time: 30 minutes | Serves 2

- 1 stalk lemongrass, bottom 6 inches only, outer leaves peeled
- 1 teaspoon extra-virgin olive oil
- 2 cloves garlic, minced
- 2 tablespoons minced shallot
- ½ cup chopped red bell pepper
- 1 cup cubed and peeled eggplant
- 1 teaspoon ground cardamom
- 1 teaspoon ground coriander
- ½ teaspoon ground cinnamon
- ½ cup canned no-salt-added diced tomatoes and their juices
- ½ cup black rice
- ⅔ cup canned "lite" coconut milk
- 1 (15-ounce) can small white beans, rinsed and drained
- 2 cups chopped baby kale
- ½ lime
- hot sauce (optional)
- salt and freshly ground black pepper (optional)

1. Lightly pound the lemongrass stalk with a kitchen mallet.
2. In a large pot, heat the olive oil over high heat. Add the garlic and shallot and cook until soft, 3 to 5 minutes. Add the bell pepper and eggplant and continue cooking until softened, 3 to 5 minutes.
3. Add the cardamom, coriander, and cinnamon and cook for 1 more minute, stirring occasionally to prevent the spices from burning.
4. Add the tomatoes, black rice, coconut milk, 1½ cups water, and beans and stir to combine. Cover, bring to a boil, then reduce the heat to low and allow to simmer for 20 minutes.
5. Stir in the kale, cover, and continue cooking until the kale is wilted, the rice is done, and most of the liquid is absorbed, 5 to 8 minutes longer.
6. To serve, remove the lemongrass stalk and squeeze in the lime juice. If desired, season with hot sauce and a dash of salt and black pepper.

PER SERVING

Calories: 433 | Total fat: 9 g | Saturated fat: 5 g | Cholesterol: 0 mg | Sodium: 32 mg | Potassium: 474 mg | Total carbohydrates: 75 g | Fiber: 16 g | Sugars: 6 g | Protein: 19 g

Lentil Bolognese

Prep time:10 minutes | Cook time: 20 minutes | Serves 4

- ¾ cup red lentils
- 2 teaspoons olive oil
- 1 onion, chopped
- 1 cup sliced mushrooms
- 2 cloves garlic, minced
- 1 carrot, grated
- 1 teaspoon dried italian seasoning
- 3 cups low-sodium vegetable broth
- ½ cup dry red wine (optional)
- 8 ounces brown rice pasta or quinoa spaghetti
- 1 (14-ounce) can no-salt-added diced tomatoes, drained
- 1 (8-ounce) can no-salt-added tomato sauce
- 2 tablespoons chopped fresh basil

1. Sort the lentils and rinse them, then set aside.
2. Heat the olive oil in a large skillet over medium-high heat. Add the onion, mushrooms, and garlic, and cook for 2 minutes, stirring frequently.
3. Add the carrot, Italian seasoning, lentils, vegetable broth, and red wine (if using), and bring to a simmer.
4. Reduce the heat to low and cook, partially covered and stirring often, for 18 to 20 minutes or until the lentils are soft.
5. Meanwhile, bring a large pot of water to a boil, add the pasta, and cook until al dente. Drain and set aside.
6. When the lentils are soft, add the tomatoes and the tomato sauce and simmer for 2 to 3 minutes. Serve the lentil sauce over the cooked spaghetti, topped with the fresh basil.

PER SERVING

Calories: 429 | Fat: 4g | Saturated Fat: 1g | Monounsaturated Fat: 2g | Carbs: 79g | Sodium: 97mg | Dietary Fiber: 16g | Protein: 18g | Cholesterol: 1mg | Vitamin A: 75% DV | Vitamin C: 37% DV | Sugar: 9g

Lentil Pilaf

Prep time:8 minutes | Cook time: 22 minutes | Serves 4

- 1¼ cup puy lentils
- 1 tablespoon olive oil
- 1 leek, white and light green parts, rinsed and chopped
- 8 ounces sliced cremini mushrooms
- 1 bay leaf
- 2 carrots, sliced
- 1½ cups frozen corn
- 3½ cups low-sodium vegetable broth
- 2 tablespoons chopped fresh basil
- 1 tablespoon minced fresh chives

1. Sort through the lentils to remove any small stones (often found in beans and lentils from the harvesting process). In a colander, rinse and drain the lentils, and set aside.
2. Heat the olive oil in a large saucepan over medium heat. Add the leeks, mushrooms, bay leaf, carrots, and corn, and cook for 2 minutes, stirring frequently.
3. Stir in the lentils and the broth and bring to a simmer. Reduce the heat to low, cover the pan, and simmer for 20 minutes or until the lentils are tender.
4. Remove from the heat and discard the bay leaf. Stir in the fresh basil and chives and serve.

PER SERVING

Calories: 348 | Fat: 6g | Saturated Fat: 1g | Monounsaturated Fat: 3g | Carbs: 59g | Sodium: 166mg | Dietary Fiber: 11g | Protein: 19g | Cholesterol: 0mg | Vitamin A: 115% DV | Vitamin C: 17% DV | Sugar: 7g

Chapter 12

Desserts

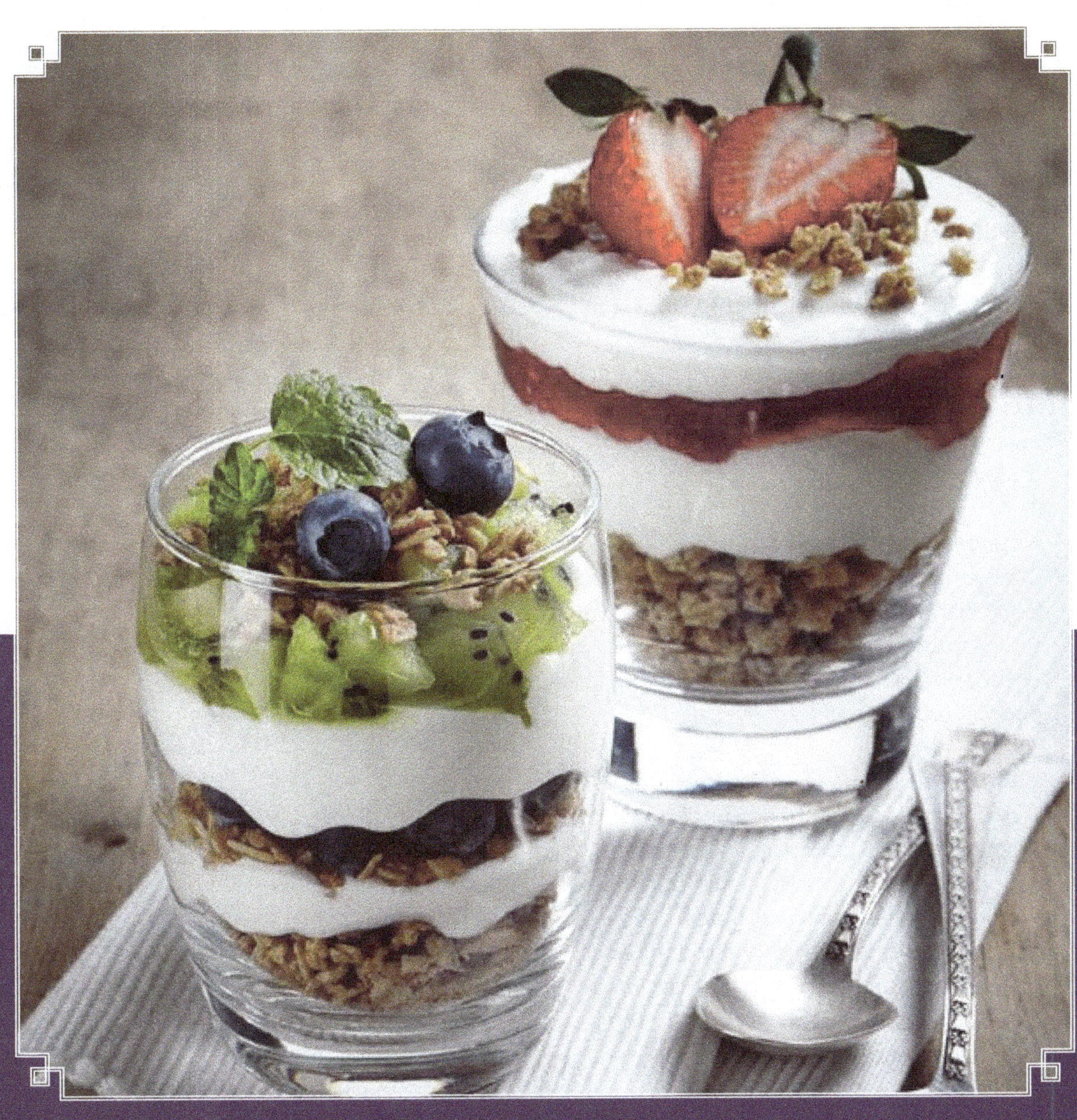

Cookies and Cream Shake

Prep time: 15 minutes | Cook time: 15 minutes | Serves 3

- 6 crushed chocolate wafer cookies,
- 3 cups of vanilla ice cream; fat-free
- 1 1/3 cups of chilled vanilla soy milk; (soya milk),

1. Combine ice cream and soy milk in a blender.
2. Blend until the mixture is smooth and foamy.
3. Toss in the cookies and pulse a few times to combine.
4. Immediately pour into tall, cold glasses and serve.

PER SERVING

Calories: 270 kcal | Protein: 9g | Carbohydrates: 52g | Fat: 3g | Cholesterol: traces | Fiber: 1 g

Honey Ricotta with Espresso and Chocolate Chips

Prep time: 5 minutes | Cook time: 15 minutes | Serves 2

- 8 ounces ricotta cheese
- 2 tablespoons honey
- 2 tablespoons espresso, chilled or room temperature
- 1 teaspoon dark chocolate chips or chocolate shavings

1. In a medium bowl, whip together the ricotta cheese and honey until light and smooth, 4 to 5 minutes.
2. Spoon the ricotta cheese–honey mixture evenly into 2 dessert bowls. Drizzle 1 tablespoon espresso into each dish and sprinkle with chocolate chips or shavings.

PER SERVING

Calories: 235 | Total fat: 10g | Saturated fat: 6g | Cholesterol: 35mg | Sodium: 115mg | Potassium: 170mg | Total Carbohydrates: 25g | Fiber: 0g | Sugars: 19g | Protein: 13g | Magnesium: 30mg | Calcium: 310mg

Gingered Asparagus

Prep time: 5 minutes | Cook time: 6 minutes | Serves 1

- ½ tablespoon fresh ginger, minced
- ½ teaspoon cumin seeds
- 1 teaspoon fresh lemon juice
- 2 tablespoons olive oil
- ½ asparagus, trimmed and cut into 2-inch pieces
- Pinch of salt
- Fresh ground black pepper to taste

1. Take a frying-pan and heat oil over medium heat and fry cumin seeds for about a minute.
2. Add remaining ingredients and stir fry for about four to five minutes.
3. Serve warm and enjoy!

PER SERVING

Calories: 268 | Fat: 28.5g | Sat Fat: 4.1g | Carbohydrates: 5.1g | Fiber: 1.9g | Sugar: 1.5g | Protein: 2g

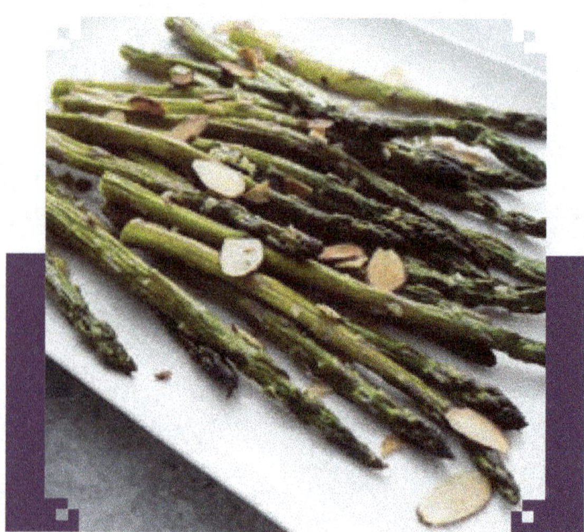

Figs with Mascarpone and Honey

Prep time: 5 minutes | Cook time: 5 minutes | Serves 4

- ⅓ cup walnuts, chopped
- 8 fresh figs, halved
- ¼ cup mascarpone cheese
- 1 tablespoon honey
- ¼ teaspoon flaked sea salt

1. In a skillet over medium heat, toast the walnuts, stirring often, 3 to 5 minutes.
2. Arrange the figs cut-side up on a plate or platter. Using your finger, make a small depression in the cut side of each fig and fill with mascarpone cheese. Sprinkle with a bit of the walnuts, drizzle with the honey, and add a tiny pinch of sea salt.

PER SERVING

Calories: 200 | Total fat: 13g | Saturated fat: 4g | Cholesterol: 18mg | Sodium: 105mg | Potassium: 230mg | Total Carbohydrates: 24g | Fiber: 3g | Sugars: 18g | Protein: 3g | Magnesium: 30mg | Calcium: 53mg

Sweet & Refreshing Sorbet

Prep time: 10 minutes | Cook time: 5 minutes | Serves 4

- ¼ cup pineapple chunks
- ¼ cup orange juice
- ½ tsp lemon juice
- ½ cup raspberries
- ½ cup strawberries
- 3 cups peaches, peeled& sliced

1. Add all ingredients into the blender and blend until smooth.
2. Pour the blended mixture into the air-tight container, cover, and place in the freezer for 6 hours.

3. Serve chilled and enjoy.

PER SERVING

Calories: 72 | Fat:0.5 g | Carbohydrates: 17.1 g | Sugar: 14.5 g | Protein: 1.5 g | Cholesterol: 0 mg

Braised Cabbage

Prep time: 5 minutes | Cook time: 30 minutes | Serves 1

- 1 garlic clove, minced
- 1½ cup green cabbage, chopped
- ¾ teaspoon olive oil
- ½ cup low-sodium vegetable broth
- ½ onion, sliced thinly
- Fresh ground black pepper to taste

1. Take a large frying pan, heat oil over medium-high heat and fry garlic for about a minute.
2. Add onion and fry for about four to five minutes.
3. Add cabbage and fry for about three to four minutes.
4. Stir in broth and black pepper and immediately, reduce the heat to low.
5. Cook while covered for about 20 minutes.
6. Serve warm and enjoy!

PER SERVING

Calories: 90 | Fat: 3.7g | Sat Fat: 0.5g | Carbohydrates: 12.8g | Fiber: 3.9g | Sugar: 5.7g | Protein: 3.2g

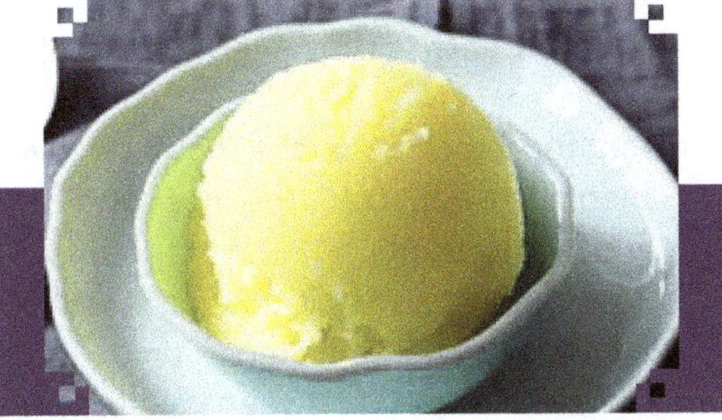

Roast Mushrooms

Prep time: 10 minutes | Cook time: 30 minutes | Serves 4

- 2 tablespoons olive oil
- 10 ounces Pink oyster mushrooms
- Black pepper to taste
- 1 teaspoon fresh basil, chopped
- 1 teaspoon fresh thyme, finely chopped
- 1 sprig rosemary
- 2 tablespoons garlic, finely sliced

1. Preheat the oven to 400° F. Oil a baking tray, add all the ingredients except the garlic to the tray.
2. Toss well to coat the mushrooms fully.
3. Roast in the oven for about 25 minutes.
4. Remove from the oven, layer the garlic beneath the mushrooms, and roast for 5 minutes.
5. Serve hot and enjoy.

PER SERVING

Calories: 94 | Fat: 7g | Sodium: 253mg | Carbs: 5g | Fiber: 2g | Sugar: 3g | Protein: 5g

Broccoli Black Bean Rice

Prep time: 10 minutes | Cook time: 30 minutes | Serves 4

- 1 cup broccoli florets, chopped
- 1 cup canned black beans, no-salt-added, drained
- 1 cup brown rice
- 2 cups low-sodium chicken stock
- 2 teaspoons sweet paprika
- Black pepper to taste

1. Put the stock in a pot, heat up over medium heat, add the rice and the other ingredients.
2. Toss, bring to a boil and cook for 30 minutes stirring from time to time.
3. Divide the mix between plates and serve as a side dish.

PER SERVING

Calories: 347 | Fat: 1.2g | Sodium: 83mg | Carbs: 69.3g | Fiber: 9g | Sugar: 1.5g | Protein: 15.1g

Zucchini Pizza Bites

Prep time: 5 minutes | Cook time: 10 minutes | Serves 1

- 1tbsp. of quick marinara sauce
- olive oil spray
- slices of large zucchini; 1/4" thick, /1 medium diagonally cut zucchini.
- 1/4 cup of part-skim shredded mozzarella
- salt and pepper

1. Cut zucchini into 1/4-inch-thick slices.
2. Season both sides with pepper and salt after gently spraying with oil.
3. Cook the zucchini for 2 minutes on each side on the broiler or the grill, and Broil for a further minute or two after topping with the cheese and sauce. (Be careful not to overcook the cheese.)

PER SERVING

Calories: 124.8 kcal | Protein: 8.2g | Carbohydrates: 10.4g | Fat: 5.7g | Cholesterol: 12mg | Fiber: 1.8g

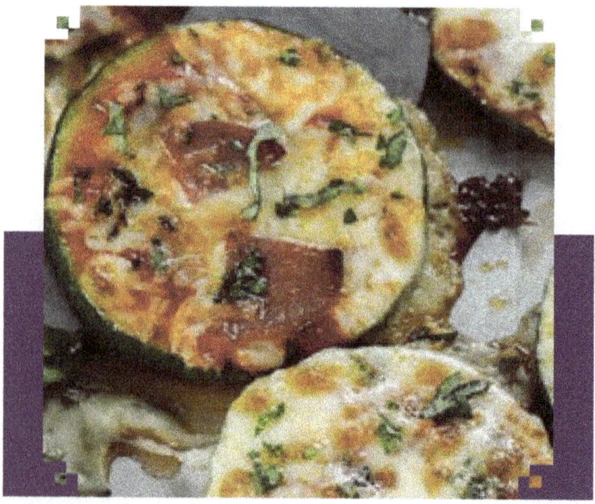

Chocolate Yogurt

Prep time: 5 minutes | Cook time: 5 minutes | Serves 1

- 1 cup Greek yogurt
- 1 tbsp unsweetened soy milk
- 1 tsp maple syrup
- 2 tbsp unsweetened cocoa powder

1. Add all ingredients into the blender and blend until smooth.
2. Pour blended mixture into the air-tight container, cover, and place in the freezer for 3 hours.
3. Serve chilled and enjoy.

PER SERVING

Calories: 200 | Fat:5.7 g | Carbohydrates: 19.8 g | Sugar: 14 g | Protein: 22.4 g | Cholesterol: 10 mg

Garlicky Broccoli

Prep time: 5 minutes | Cook time: 8 minutes | Serves 1

- ½ tablespoon olive oil
- 1 cup broccoli florets
- 1 tablespoon water
- 1 garlic clove, minced
- Fresh ground black pepper to taste
- Pinch of salt

1. Take a large frying pan, heat the oil over medium heat and fry the garlic for about a minute.
2. Add the broccoli and stir fry for two minutes.
3. Stir in water, salt and black pepper and stir fry for four to five minutes.
4. Carefully open each parcel and serve hot.

PER SERVING

Calories: 96 | Fat: 7.3g | Sat Fat: 1g | Carbohydrates:

7.1g | Fiber: 2.5g | Sugar: 1.6g | Protein: 2.8g

Roasted Plums with Nut Crumble

Prep time: 5 minutes | Cook time: 25 minutes | Serves 4

- ¼ cup honey
- ¼ cup freshly squeezed orange juice
- 4 large plums, halved and pitted
- ¼ cup whole-wheat pastry flour
- 1 tablespoon pure maple sugar
- 1 tablespoon nuts, coarsely chopped (your choice; I like almonds, pecans, and walnuts)
- 1½ teaspoons canola oil
- ½ cup plain Greek yogurt

1. Preheat the oven to 400°F. Combine the honey and orange juice in a square baking dish. Place the plums, cut-side down, in the dish. Roast about 15 minutes, and then turn the plums over and roast an additional 10 minutes, or until tender and juicy.
2. In a medium bowl, combine the flour, maple sugar, nuts, and canola oil and mix well. Spread on a small baking sheet and bake alongside the plums, tossing once, until golden brown, about 5 minutes. Set aside until the plums have finished cooking.
3. Serve the plums drizzled with pan juices and topped with the nut crumble and a dollop of yogurt.

PER SERVING

Calories: 175 | Total fat: 3g | Saturated fat: 0g | Cholesterol: 0mg | Sodium: 10mg | Potassium: 215mg | Total Carbohydrates: 36g | Fiber: 2g | Sugars: 28g | Protein: 4g | Magnesium: 22mg | Calcium: 40mg

Appendix 1 Measurement Conversion Chart

Volume Equivalents (Dry)

US STANDARD	METRIC (APPROXIMATE)
1/8 teaspoon	0.5 mL
1/4 teaspoon	1 mL
1/2 teaspoon	2 mL
3/4 teaspoon	4 mL
1 teaspoon	5 mL
1 tablespoon	15 mL
1/4 cup	59 mL
1/2 cup	118 mL
3/4 cup	177 mL
1 cup	235 mL
2 cups	475 mL
3 cups	700 mL
4 cups	1 L

Volume Equivalents (Liquid)

US STANDARD	US STANDARD (OUNCES)	METRIC (APPROXIMATE)
2 tablespoons	1 fl.oz.	30 mL
1/4 cup	2 fl.oz.	60 mL
1/2 cup	4 fl.oz.	120 mL
1 cup	8 fl.oz.	240 mL
1 1/2 cup	12 fl.oz.	355 mL
2 cups or 1 pint	16 fl.oz.	475 mL
4 cups or 1 quart	32 fl.oz.	1 L
1 gallon	128 fl.oz.	4 L

Temperatures Equivalents

FAHRENHEIT(F)	CELSIUS(C) APPROXIMATE
225 °F	107 °C
250 °F	120 ° °C
275 °F	135 °C
300 °F	150 °C
325 °F	160 °C
350 °F	180 °C
375 °F	190 °C
400 °F	205 °C
425 °F	220 °C
450 °F	235 °C
475 °F	245 °C
500 °F	260 °C

Weight Equivalents

US STANDARD	METRIC (APPROXIMATE)
1 ounce	28 g
2 ounces	57 g
5 ounces	142 g
10 ounces	284 g
15 ounces	425 g
16 ounces (1 pound)	455 g
1.5 pounds	680 g
2 pounds	907 g

Appendix 2 The Dirty Dozen and Clean Fifteen

The Environmental Working Group (EWG) is a nonprofit, nonpartisan organization dedicated to protecting human health and the environment Its mission is to empower people to live healthier lives in a healthier environment. This organization publishes an annual list of the twelve kinds of produce, in sequence, that have the highest amount of pesticide residue-the Dirty Dozen-as well as a list of the fifteen kinds ofproduce that have the least amount of pesticide residue-the Clean Fifteen.

THE DIRTY DOZEN	
The 2016 Dirty Dozen includes the following produce. These are considered among the year's most important produce to buy organic:	
Strawberries	Spinach
Apples	Tomatoes
Nectarines	Bell peppers
Peaches	Cherry tomatoes
Celery	Cucumbers
Grapes	Kale/collard greens
Cherries	Hot peppers
The Dirty Dozen list contains two additional itemskale/collard greens and hot peppers-because they tend to contain trace levels of highly hazardous pesticides.	

THE CLEAN FIFTEEN	
The least critical to buy organically are the Clean Fifteen list. The following are on the 2016 list:	
Avocados	Papayas
Corn	Kiw
Pineapples	Eggplant
Cabbage	Honeydew
Sweet peas	Grapefruit
Onions	Cantaloupe
Asparagus	Cauliflower
Mangos	
Some of the sweet corn sold in the United States are made from genetically engineered (GE) seedstock. Buy organic varieties of these crops to avoid GE produce.	

Appendix 3 Index

Robin K. Solis

www.ingramcontent.com/pod-product-compliance
Lightning Source LLC
Chambersburg PA
CBHW082213231025
34481CB00012B/564